Artur Broclawski,
Solmaz Golsabahi-Broclawski (Eds.)
Marianne Kastrup, Ibrahim Özkan,
Hans Rohlof, Ron Wintrob (Co-Eds.)

Transcultural Challenge of Medicine

Schriftenreihe zur transkulturellen Psychiatrie, Psychotherapie und Psychosomatik

herausgegeben von

Solmaz Golsabahi-Broclawski

Band 7

LIT

Transcultural Challenge of Medicine

First International Conference on Transcultural Psychiatry in Central European Countries

edited by

Artur Broclawski
and Solmaz Golsabahi-Broclawski

Marianne Kastrup, Ibrahim Özkan,
Hans Rohlof, Ron Wintrob (Co-Eds.)

LIT

This book is printed on acid-free paper.

Bibliographic information published by the Deutsche Nationalbibliothek
The Deutsche Nationalbibliothek lists this publication in the Deutsche Nationalbibliografie; detailed bibliographic data are available on the Internet at http://dnb.d-nb.de.

ISBN 978-3-643-90744-8

A catalogue record for this book is available from the British Library

Klosbachstr. 107
CH-8032 Zürich
Tel. +41 (0) 44-251 75 05
E-Mail: zuerich@lit-verlag.ch http://www.lit-verlag.ch
Distribution:
In the UK: Global Book Marketing, e-mail: mo@centralbooks.com
In North America: International Specialized Book Services, e-mail: orders@isbs.com
In Germany: LIT Verlag Fresnostr. 2, D-48159 Münster
Tel. +49 (0) 2 51-620 32 22, Fax +49 (0) 2 51-922 60 99, e-mail: vertrieb@lit-verlag.de
In Austria: Medienlogistik Pichler-ÖBZ, e-mail: mlo@medien-logistik.at
e-books are available at www.litwebshop.de

Contents

Foreword

First International Conference on Transcultural Psychiatry in Central European Countries

Gdynia, Poland, 24–26 April 2015

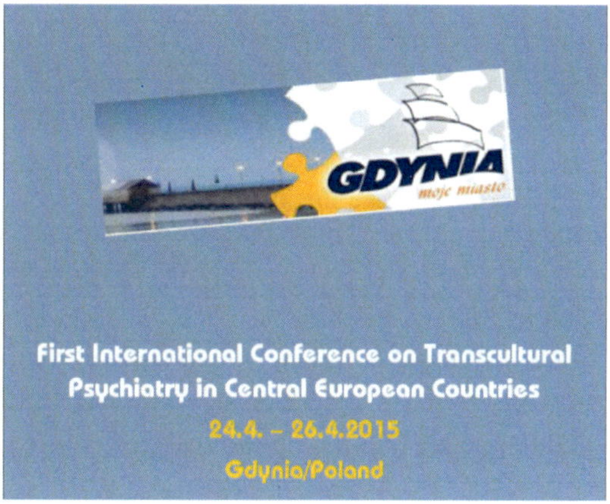

Sponsoring Organizations

MITK (www.mitk.eu), WPA-TPS (www.wpa-tps.org) in cooperation with DTPPP (www.dtppp.com)

Organizing Committee

Marianne Kastrup (WPA-TPS), Artur Broclawski (MITK), Solmaz Golsabahi-Broclawski (MITK, DTPPP), Hans Rohlof (WPA-TPS), Ron Wintrob (WPA-TPS)

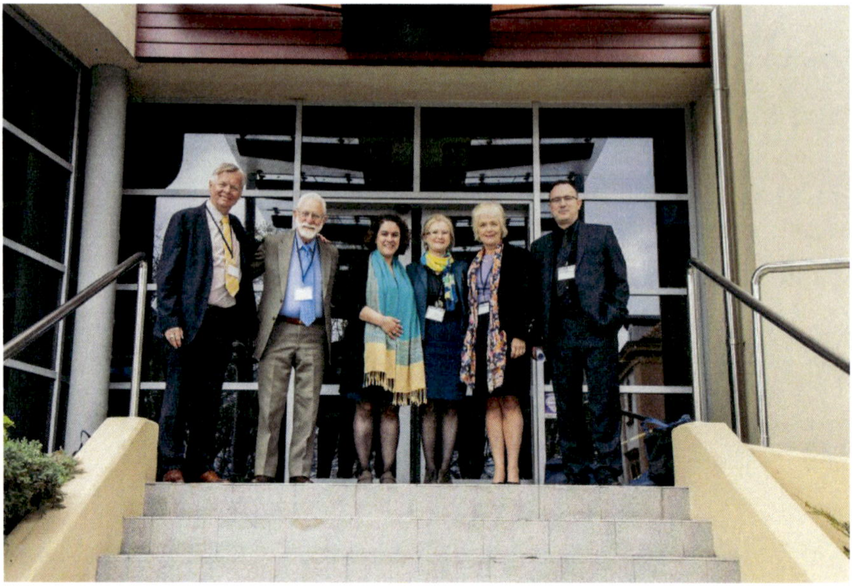

Picture 24.4.2015 Gdynia, Poland: Hans Rohlof, Ron Wintrob, Solmaz Golsabahi-Broclawski, Ljiliana Joksimovic, Marianne Kastrup, Artur Broclawski

Dear Colleagues,

We want to inform you with this newsletter about the current activities of our Institute in the field of cross-cultural psychiatry and transcultural medicine. As you are aware, the association of German- speaking transcultural psychiatry, psychotherapy and psychosomatic (DTPPP e.V), which was inaugurated in 2007, has organised annual congresses related to culture and mental health services and has become a platform for interpersonal contact and sharing experiences among contributors to research and clinical care in this field.

Dr. Golsabahi- Broclawski, who is one of the founders of the association and was the chair of DTPP from 2007 through 2014, is now responsible for networking of the association. She has chaired the Organizing Committee for the conference in Gdynia, in coordination with Artur Broclawski, Marianne Kastrup, Hans Rohlof and Ron Wintrob. The Mayor of Gdynia, Mr. Szczurek is the official patronal of the Conference and Prof. Landowski, the chief director of the psychiatry Department of the University of Gdy-

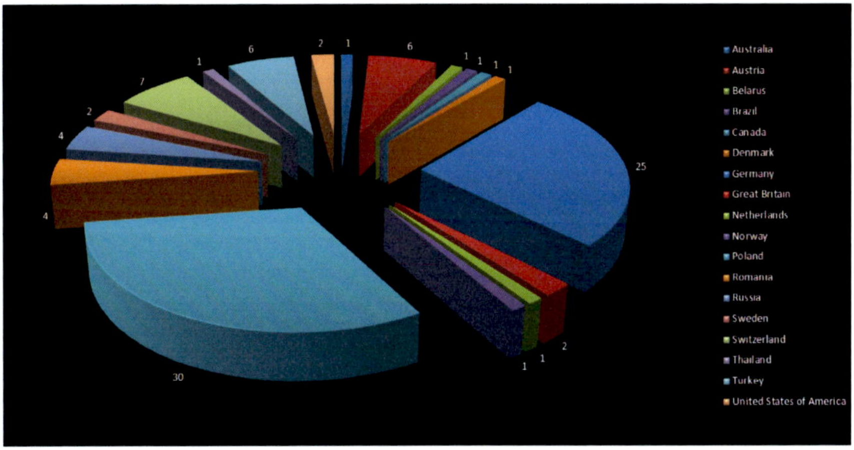

nia is our cooperation partner from Poland. This conference has developed from other collaborative efforts between DTPPP, WPA-TPS and EPA, beginning with the conference on sharing experiences of transcultural psychiatry in Europe, held in Hamm, Germany in February 2012.

This First International Conference on Transcultural Psychiatry in Central European Countries, held in Gdynia, Poland, in April 2015, attracted the participation of 110 colleagues from 26 countries and 5 continents. It offered participants very good opportunities for sharing experiences and knowledge on topics such as adaptation to migration, asylum, acculturative stress and transcultural education.

The scientific program of the Conference included six thematic workshops, 12 symposia and plenary presentations comprising some 30 lectures, in addition to 10 poster presentations Topics of the conference in 2015 included:

- National Immigration Policies and Their Mental Health Implications,
- Transcultural Positive Family Therapy,
- Psychological Aspects of "Asylum shopping "
- Treatment of Migrants and Asylum Seekers

Topics of practical focus included:

- Migration and the Daily Life of Migrants,
- Best Practice Models

- Development of Cross-cultural and Transcultural Approaches in Psychotherapeutic Practice and Research
- Transcultural Balint Groups,
- Cross-cultural Supervision

Our colleagues from Russia were, unfortunately, not able to participate in the conference because of unanticipated visa problems and related circumstances. Nevertheless, their lectures will be published along with those of the other conference participants, because we want to emphasize the point that scientific concepts and their associated clinical experiences are not limited by political restrictions and will survive current obstacles in professional sharing and communication.

We will post some of the pictures from the conference on our website (www.mitk.eu) so that you can get an impression of the atmosphere of these three cordial and productive days.

Gdynia has proven to be an especially attractive location for the conference; in part, because Gdynia is an example of major community development over the past two decades, strongly influenced by the effects of migration. This part of Poland has a long history of trade with the world, and has been the locus of extensive and protracted inter-nation conflict, occupation and fight for freedom and independence during the 19th and 20th centuries. Thanks to intense migration and the dynamic growth of its commercial port over the past 20 years, Gdynia has become transformed from a fishing village into a city with international connections and a vibrant cultural life

Drawing on comments made by participants in the evaluation forms for the conference in Gdynia/2015, we plan to divide the conference in 2017 into two parts: the first part being scientific symposia and plenary sessions and the second part being a practical component focusing on the everyday work in the clinical area, including Balint group discussion, case supervision and transcultural educational lectures.

On behalf of the international Organizing Committee we want to thank Mrs Yasmin Haunold (CE-Management, Vienna). She has been responsible for the administrative organization of the DTPPP conferences since 2006, and of conferences co-sponsored by WPA-TPS and by MITK over the past several years. Her organizational and interpersonal skills have been a key component in the success of these conferences.

We will keep you informed you as planning for the program of the 'Gdynia conference/2017' proceeds, and we invite you to participate with us in the 2nd international conference on transcultural psychiatry in Gdansk and Gdynia, Poland in two years time.

All of the lectures of the conference 2015 will be published so that everyone will be able to reflect on and discuss their main points with colleagues, in anticipation of further discussion of these topics at the 'follow-up' conference to be held in 2017.

Yours

Medical Institute of transcultural competent
www.mitk.eu

A. Broclawski
S. Golsabahi-Broclawski

Pierwsza miedzynarodowa konferencja psychiatrii transkulturowej w krajach Europy środkowej

Gdynia, 24–26.04.2015

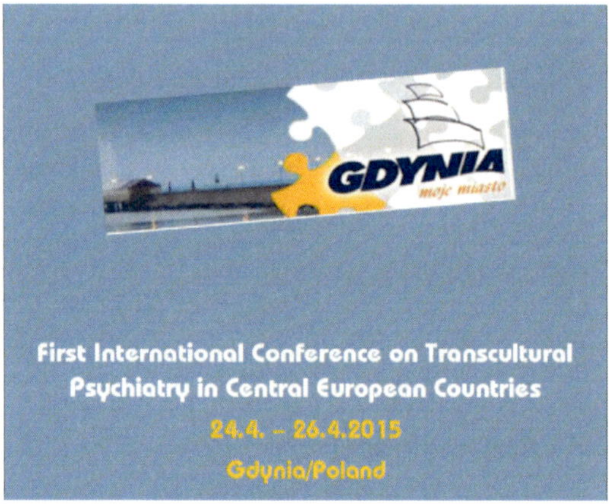

Organizatorzy konferencji:

MITK (www.mitk.eu) i WPA-tps (www.wpa-tps.org) w kooperacji z DTPPP (www.dtppp.com)

Komitet organizacyjny:

Marianne Kastrup (WPA-tps), Artur Broclawski (MItK), Solmaz Golsabhi-Broclawski (MItK, DTPP), Hans Rohlof (WPA-tps) oraz Ron Wintrob (WPA-tps)

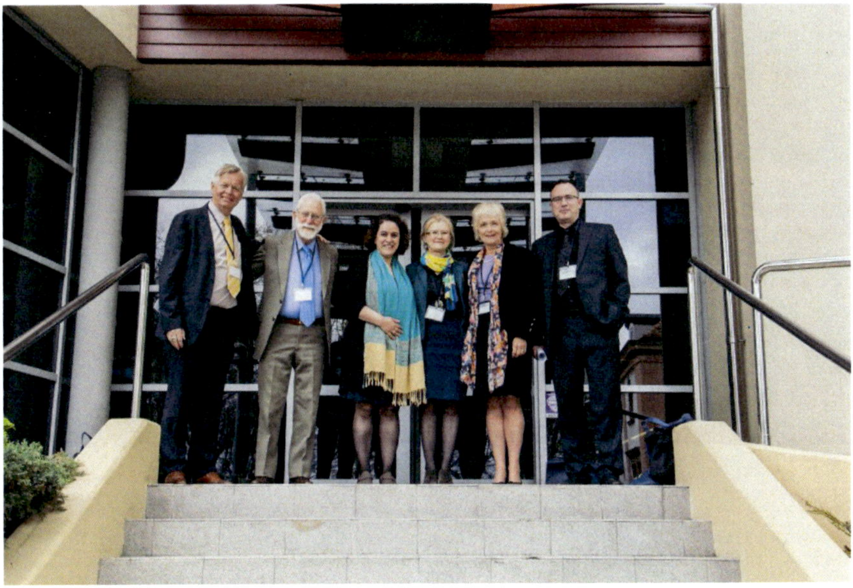

Foto: 25.04.2015 Gdynia: Od lewej: Hans Rohlof, Ron Wintrob, Solmaz Golsabhi-Broclawski, Liljana Joksimovic, Marianne Kastrup, Artur Broclawski

Szanowne koleżanki i koledzy,

za pośrednictwem tego *newsletter* chcemy Państwa informować o aktualnych przedsięwzięciach naszego instytutu na polu psychiatrie i transkulturowej medycyny. Jak Panstwu wiadomo Zrzeszenie niemieckojezycznej transkulturowej psychiatrii, psychoterapie i psychosomatyki (DTPPP e.V.), które zostało zalożone w roku 2007, organizuje od tego czasu coroczne kongresy związane z tematem transkulturowymi w ramach ochrony zdrowia psychicznego. Kongresy te stały się z czasem doskonałą okazją umożliwiającą bezpośrednie spotkania i wymianę doświadczeń na tym polu pomiędzy instytucjami, organizacjami jak i pojedyńczymi osobami.

Pani Dr. Solmaz Golsabhi-Broclawski, która była jedną z założycieli zrzeszenia (DTPP) i jego przewodniczącą (2007–2014) jest odpowiedzialna w tej organizacji za kontakty miedzynarodowe i współpracę z innymi instytucjami.

We współpracy z Arturem Brocławskim (Polska/Niemcy), Hansem

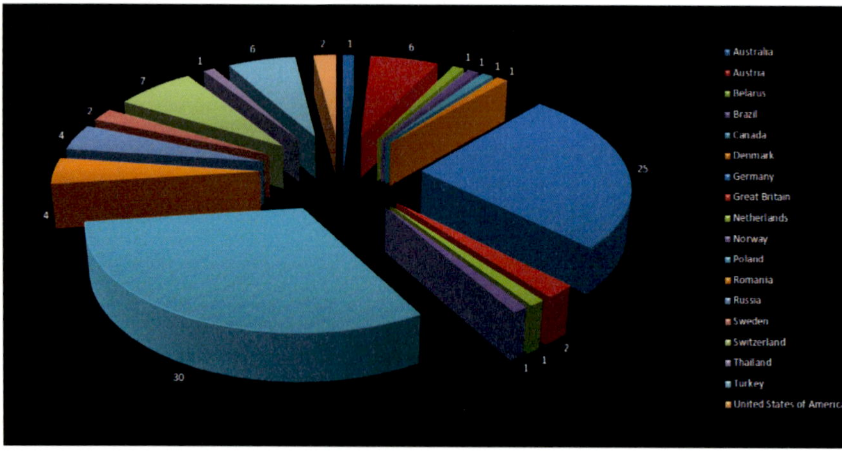

Rohlof (Holandia; honorowy były przewodniczący WPA-tps), Marianne Kastrup (Dania, aktualna przewodnicząca WPA-tps; oraz Ronem Wintrob (USA, także honorowym byłym przewodniczący WPA-tps) przewodniczyła ona komitetowi organizacyjnemu konferecji w Gdyni.

U podstaw te konferencji leżała dobra współpraca DTPPP, WPA-tps und EPA, która zaowocowała konferencją dotyczącą wymiany doświadczeń na polu psychiatrii transkulturowej w Europie w lutym 2012 w Hamm (Nadrenia-Westfalia, Niemcy).

W pierwszej międzynarodowej konferencja psychiatrii transkulturowej w krajach Europy środkowej, która odbyła się w w kwietniu 2015 w Gdyni, wziąło udzial 110 uczestników z 26 krajów i 5 kontynentów. Konferencja była świetną okazją do wymiany dośswiadczeń w zakresie migracji, asylu, uchodźców, stresu akulturowego oraz edukacji transkulturowej.

Patronat honorowy Konferencji sprawował Prezydent Miasta Gdynia, w którego imieniu konferencję otworzyła pani Teresa Marzejon, naczelnik wydziału zdrowia Miasta Gdynia.

Pan prof. Jerzy Lewandowski Kierownik Katedry Psychiatrii Uniwersytetu Medycznego w Gdansku, powitał uczestników konferecji jako przedstawiciel środowiska psychiatrycznego na Pomorzu.

Program naukowy konferencji w Gdyni skladał się z 6 warsztatów tematycznych, 12 sympozjów oraz posiedznń plenarnych wraz z 30 referatami oraz z 10 prezentacji posterowych.

Główne tematy konferencji w roku 2015 (w wersji ang.):

- National Immigration Policies and Their Mental Health Implications,
- Transcultural Positive Family Therapy,
- Psychological Aspects of "Asylum shopping "
- Treatment of Migrants and Asylum Seekers

Główne tematy części "praktycznej" (w wersji ang):

- Migration and the Daily Life of Migrants,
- Best Practice Models
- Development of Cross-cultural and Transcultural Approaches in Psychotherapeutic Practice and Research
- Transcultural Balint Groups,
- Cross-cultural Supervision

Nasi koledzy z Rosji (częściowo aż z dalekiej Syberii) z powodów problemów wizowych nie mogli wziąść bezpośredniego udziału w naszej konferencji 2015. Ich referarty będą jednakże opublikowane wraz z pozostałymi materiałami konferencji, by podkreślić, iż koncepcje naukowe oraz ich zastosowanie w praktyce klinicznej nie tylko nie są limitowane politycznymi ograniczeniami lecz są trwałym elementen profesjonalnej wymiany naukowej i komunikacji.

Materiały konferencyjne – Na naszej stronie internetowej (www.mitk.eu) zaprezentujemy wkrótce zdjęcia, które dobrze oddają koleżeńską i twórczą atmosferę konferencji.

Referaty konferencyjne zostaną wkrótce opublikowane aby umożliwić dalszą dyskusję w dalszych kręgach jako przygotowanie do nastęnej konferencji w roku 2017.

W tym miejscu chcielibyśmy też szczególnie serdecznie podziękować pani Yasmin Haunold (CE-Mangement z Wiednia). Jej organizacyjne talenty jak i osobiste zaangażowanie w konferencję były jednym z podstaw sukcesu konferencji.

Lokalizacja konferencji – miasto Gdynia okazało się atrakcyjnym miejscem an konferencję, szczególnie, iż jst ono doskonałym przykładem rozwoju miasta i jego społecznosci w kontekście zjawisk migracyjnych na przestrzeni wielu dziesięcioleci (zarówno wewnątrzkrajowych jaki i emigracyjnych). Ten rejon Polski (Pomorze) mający długą tradycję kontaktów i handlu z całym światem był równocześnie miejscem wielu międzynarodowych konfliktów, okupacji oraz walki o wolność i niepodległość w okresie ostatnich dwóch stuleci.

W ciągu 90 lat istnienia Gdynia przeistoczyła się z małej wioski rybackiej w miasto o międzynarodowych powiązaniach, pulsującym życiu kulturalnym oraz naukowym.

Następna konferencja w roku 2017 – Na gruncie intensywnej wymiany doświadczeń oraz wiedzy naukowej w tych tematach zostało jeszcze t trakcie konferencji ustalone, iż ponowna konferencja zorganizowana będzie w roku 2017, ponownie w Gdyni. Na podstawie dotychczasowach uwag i propozycji uczestników konferencji planujemy podzielić konferencję w 2017 roku na część naukowej

wymiany (sympozja oraz posiedzenia plenarne) oraz na część "praktyczną" skupiającą się na codziennej pracy klinicznej, zawierającą dyskusję w ramach grupy Balinta, superwizję oraz temat edukacji transkulturowej.

Na bieżąco będziemy informować Państwo o przebiegu przygotowań do następnej, II międzynarodowej konferencja psychiatrii transkulturowej w Gdyni w roku 2017 oraz już teraz zapraszamy do udziału w niej.

Z koleżeńskimi pozdrowieniami

A. Broclawski
S. Golsabahi-Broclawski

First International Conference on Transcultural Psychiatry in Central European Countries, Gdynia Poland

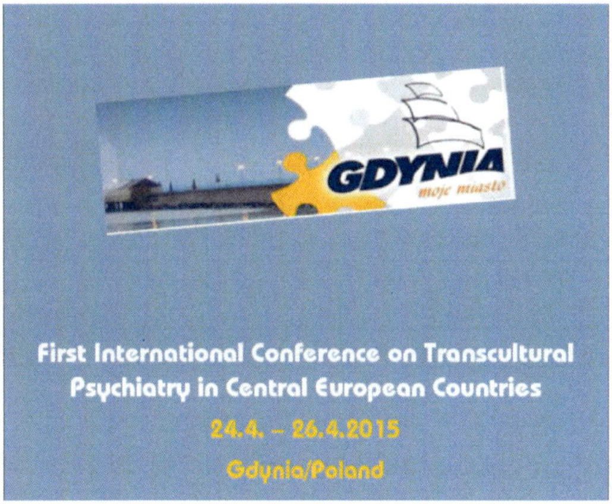

Sponsoren der Veranstaltung

MITK (www.mitk.eu), WPA-TPS(www.wpa-tps.org) in Kooperation mit DTPPP www.dtppp.com).

Veranstalter vor Ort

Marianne Kastrup (WPA-tps), Artur Broclawski (MITK), Solmaz Golsabahi-Broclawski (MITK, DTPPP), Hans Rohlof (WPA-Tps), Ron Wintrob (WPA-tps).

Liebe Kolleginnen und Kollegen,

mit diesem Newsletter werden wir Sie über unsere Aktivitäten im Bereich der transkulturellen Psychiatrie, Psychotherapie, Psychosomatik, Psychologie, Sozialarbeit, Ethnologie, Pflege und gutachterliche Bereiche auf

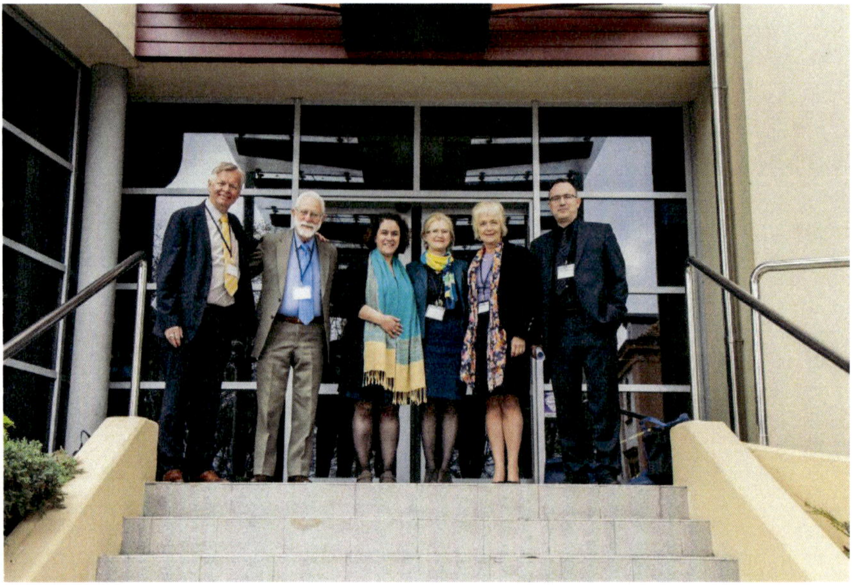

Foto 24.4.2015 Gdynia/Polen: Hans Rohlof, Ron Wintrob, Solmaz Golsabah-Broclawaski, Ljiliana Joksimovic, Marianne Kastrup, Artur Broclawski

dem Laufenden halten, um auch auf diesem Wege die Qualität unseres Faches voranzutreiben.

Wie Sie wissen, ist der Dachverband der transkulturellen Psychiatrie, Psychotherapie und Psychosomatik DTPPP e.V. bereits seit 2007 aktiv und leistet einen hervorragenden Beitrag zur Optimierung und Vernetzung der im Bereich der transkulturellen Medizin tätigen Verbände, Institutionen, Organisationen und Einzelpersonen. In diesem Rahmen hat der Dachverband mehrere Arbeitsgruppen installiert, um dieses Ziel zu erreichen.

Das Medizinische Institut der transkulturellen Medizin, gegründet 2009, und die Arbeitsgruppe *Vernetzung* der DTPPP unter der Leitung von Frau Dr. Golsabahi-Broclawski hat bereits 2012 eine enge Kooperation mit WPA-tps gestartet. Die erste Veranstaltung fand in diesem Rahmen mit Unterstützung und Realisierung von Marianne Kastrup, Hans Rohlof, Ron Wintrob in Hamm statt.

Nach langjährigem und engmaschigem Austausch der Beteiligten fand im April 2015 in Gdynia/Polen die erste gemeinsame Veranstaltung in Ko-

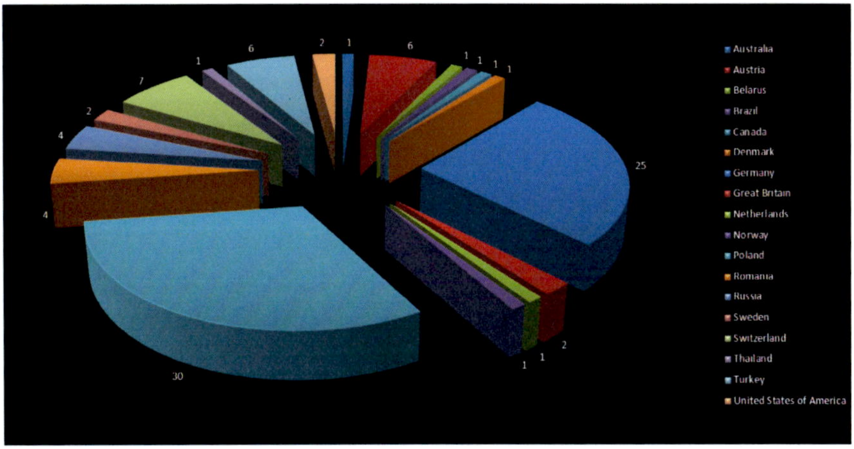

operation auf internationaler Ebene statt. An dem Kongress nahmen 110 Personen, aus 26 Ländern und 5 Kontinenten teil. In dem Rahmen kam es zu einem dreitägigen intensiven Austausch über die Themen rund um Migration, Flucht und transkulturelle Ausbildung und Erfahrung.

Die Ehrenschirmherrschaft übernahm der Bürgermeister der Stadt Gdynia Herr Szczurek und die wissenschaftliche Beratung vor Ort lief über die psychiatrische Fakultät der medizinischen Universität Danzig, Prof. Lewandowski.

Es wurden insgesamt 6 Workshops, 12 Symposien, sowie 10 Poster-Präsentationen durchgeführt, und 30 Referenten haben ihre Erfahrungen aus dem Bereich der Praxis und Forschung vorgetragen.

Besonders hervorzuheben sind an dieser Stelle die Beiträge zu den Themen:

- National Immigration Policies and Their Mental Health Implications,
- Transcultural Positive Family Therapy,
- Psychological Aspects of "Asylum shopping"
- Treatment of Migrants and Asylum Seekers

sowie die klinisch relevanten Beiträge zu den Themen:

- Migration and the Daily Life of Migrants,
- Best Practice Models

- Development of Cross-cultural and Transcultural Approaches in Psychotherapeutic Practice and Research
- Transcultural Balint Group
- Cross-cultural Supervision

Die Kollegen aus Russland und Sibirien haben leider kurzfristig aus politischen und einreisespezifischen Gründen keine Einreiseerlaubnis erhalten. Wir bedauern dies sehr und gleichzeitig vergegenwärtigt uns diese Tatsache die enorme Präsens und Aktualität der angesprochenen Themen. Die Kollegen aus Moskau, Sibirien und Ukraine werden nichtsdestotrotz ihre Beiträge in schriftlicher Form einreichen, damit sie einerseits durch die Publikation Gehör finden und andererseits ein Zeichen zu setzen, dass die Wissenschaft und Forschung die Politik überdauern wird.

Wir werden Ihnen eine Bilderreihe auf der Homepage www.mitk.eu erstellen, damit Sie einen persönlichen Eindruck von der dortigen Atmosphäre erhalten.

Der Ort des Kongresses wurde seitens des Medizinischen Institutes für transkulturelle Kompetenz ganz geziehlt ausgesucht: Gdynia ist ein Ort an der Küste Polens, den es nur dank der Migrationspolitik und aufgrund der Migrationsströmungen des 19. Jahrhunderts gibt und wo die Menschen aus allen Bereichen des damaligen Polens versucht haben, sich dort eine neue Zukunft zu schaffen. Viele haben auch zu unterschiedlichen Zeitpunkten der Geschichte von dort aus die Flucht übers Meer unternommen, um sich vor politischen Verfolgungen zu retten und eine neue Zukunft aufzubauen. Nach einer Auswertung der Evaluationen wurde seitens der Veranstalter beschlossen, den internationalen transkulturellen Psychiatrie Kongress 2017 in Gdynia aufzuteilen in einen wissenschaftlichen Austauschbereich und einen Bereich relevant für den praktisch-klinischen Alltag mit Balint-Gruppen, Supervision und interkulturelle Trainingseinheiten für Interessierte und Einsteiger im Bereich der transkulturellen Medizin.

An dieser Stelle möchten wir uns ganz herzlich bei Frau Yasmin Haunold (CE-Management Wien) bedanken. Dank ihrer transkulturellen Fertigkeiten ermöglicht Ihr Team die Zusammenkunft und Organisation auf der Handlungsebene der unterschiedlichen Wissenschaftler und klinisch tätigen Kollegen aus aller Welt.

Wir werden Sie einmal im Quartal über die Aktivitäten informieren und freuen uns auf Ihre Impulse zur Optimierung der Vernetzung des Austausches auf internationaler Ebene.

Die Publikation der vorgetragenen Beiträge wird demnächst auf der Homepage www.mitk.eu sowie per Rundmail der DTPPP e.V. bekanntgegeben.

Ihr

Medizinisches Institut für transkulturelle Kompetenz

A. Broclawski
S. Golsabahi-Broclawski

Culture, Medicine and the Future of Person-centered Treatment

Ronald Wintrob MD

Introduction: Scope, Dimensions and Topics of Research in Transcultural Psychiatry; Historical Perspective

In 1969, the American Psychiatric Association and the Canadian Psychiatric Association endorsed and published a position statement formulated by the Transcultural Psychiatry committees of the two organizations.

The position statement defined transcultural psychiatry as the comparative study of mental health and mental illness among different societies, nations and cultures, and the inter-relationships of mental disorders with cultural environments (American Psychiatric Association, Committee on Transcultural Psychiatry, 1969).

The position statement indicated that clinical service and research in transcultural psychiatry should focus on the following key issues;

- the understanding of conflict in persons experiencing rapid social and cultural change
- the psychological and social adaptation of both voluntary and involuntary migrants within, as well as across, national boundaries
- cultural determinants of public policy decisions within and between nations, including their implications for the mental health of indigenous, minority and immigrant components of national populations.

Furthermore, it was recommended that research in transcultural psychiatry should take careful account of how human beings think, feel and act, with reference to the sociocultural contexts in which they are reared or live as adults, including both subjectively experienced states and objectively observable behavior, whether defined as normal, sick or deviant.

The position statement included twelve main areas for research, including;

- Similarities and differences in the form, course, or manifestation of mental illness in different societies and cultures
- The occurrence, incidence and distribution of mental illness or behavioral characteristics in relation to sociocultural factors
- Sociocultural factors predisposing to mental illness or to optimal function, or increasing vulnerability to impaired function
- The forms of treatment and prevention that are preferred in various sociocultural settings
- The influence of sociocultural factors on the diagnosis, treatment and prevention of mental illness
- The understanding of conflict in persons experiencing rapid social and cultural change
- Attitudes and beliefs regarding the labeling of behavior as deviant or mentally ill
- The psychological and social adaptation of voluntary or involuntary migrants within or across national boundaries
- Cultural determinants of transnational interactions, and of public policy decisions within and between nations

It was noted that specific research projects would require the involvement of individuals, families and groups from differing nations, social classes or ethnic groups, and of those subscribing to different values and belief systems within the majority culture. Furthermore, research in transcultural psychiatry needed to include people who share fully in the values and opportunities of their society as members of the majority group, as well as those who are excluded or bypassed from full participation by their being members of indigenous minority groups, immigrants and members of racially, ethnically and religiously distinct minority groups within national populations.

Global Migration: The Political, Demographic, Social and Mental Health Implications of Steadily Increasing International Migration

Once again nations around the world are experiencing an era of unanticipated, rapid increase in migration. The scale of such migration and the desperate situation of millions of migrants swept up in both intra-national and inter-national conflict, seem to have overwhelmed the capacity of receiving nations to cope with the inflow of migrants.

Not only are few nations willing and able to provide security and opportunity for these migrants, but in many receiving nations a backlash of resentment and hostility toward migrants has greatly added to the anxiety, mutual alienation and fear for their safety among both migrants and people of the receiving nations. The risks for deterioration of the social cohesion and the mental health of both host and migrant populations under these very stressful conditions are all too apparent.

From 1990 to 2010, the number of migrants in the world has increased from 150 to 200 million people. Migrants in Europe increased from 50 to 68 million, comprising >10% of the total European population. By 2005, the number of migrants in Germany, France, Spain, UK, Netherlands and several other European countries had reached or exceeded 15% of their national populations.

All of these numbers have continued to rise steadily since 2010, and the waves of migrants from war-torn countries of the Middle East, Asia and Africa have endured perilous journeys to land on the shores and cross the hills and forests of many European countries in search of safety, hope and opportunity.

By 2005, migrants in Australia – a country that only ended its official "White Australia" immigration policy in the 1980s – comprised 20% of the national population.

In response to similar circumstances, migrant numbers in North America from 1990 to 2010 have increased from 28 to 50 million; 15% of the total North American population. By 2005, the number of ('documented') immigrants in the USA exceeded 36 million people; 13% of the national population. In addition, there are approximately 12 million 'undocumented' (illegal) migrants living in the USA.

The annual report of the United Nations High Commission on Refugees, published in June, 2014, indicated that by the end of 2013, the number of refugees in the world exceeded 51 million people; the highest number since WW2 (United Nations High Commission on Refugees, 2014). A year later, the number of refugees in the world reached 59.5 million (United Nations High Commission for Refugees, 2015). These figures represent an increase of 22 million people displaced as refugees since 2005, due to war, internal national conflicts, persecution and forced migration. In 2014 alone, the number of refugees rose by 8.3 million; the largest yearly increase in the 50 years that UNHCR has been monitoring refugee numbers. By the end of 2014, 1 out of every 122 people in the world was a refugee; either internally displaced in their home country, or actively seeking asylum in another country. Most alarmingly, over half of all refugees are children, an increasing number of them unaccompanied by any family members. In 2013 alone, 11 million people were newly displaced. Eighty-six % of refugees in the world are living in 'low income' countries; a much higher proportion than 10 years ago. In Europe, there was an overall increase in refugees of 51% in 2014. The 2015 UNHCR report projects an even greater increase in refugee numbers in the year ahead. In 2013, 414,000 refugees were able to return to their home countries. In 2014, that number dropped sharply; to 127,000. Less than 100,000 refugees were accepted for resettlement as immigrants by other countries in 2013 and in 2014. In 2013, 1.1 million people applied for asylum status in other countries, the highest number in a decade.

The unprecedented humanitarian crisis that these statistics represent has generated equally unprecedented political, legal, social, medical and psychiatric service dilemmas for receiving nations around the world. The scale of the crisis has, so far, overwhelmed the innate humanitarian instincts and available resources of help in receiving nations everywhere.

Implications of Increased Migration and Resettlement for Cultural Diversity and Multiculturalism

Many countries that had been ethnically homogeneous before 1980 became culturally diverse. This has not only been evident in Europe, North America and Australia, but also in many countries in Asia, South America and Africa. There has also been massive rural to urban migration that has created numerous mega-cities throughout Asia, Africa and Latin America. Steadily increasing cultural diversity and multiculturalism have been reflected in the changing demographic composition of health care and social service facilities in migration-affected countries everywhere – as well as parallel changes in schools and judicial services. The need for countries to recognize and take account of a new cultural diversity in their national populations has profoundly affected the life of cities, regions and countries that had not paid much attention to the national implications of burgeoning multiculturalism in decades past.

Changes in the demographic composition of the USA population since 1980 are a powerful illustration of the impact of steadily increasing immigration leading to much greater ethnic diversity and a new multiculturalist way of life – despite some surges of resentment, anti-immigrant sentiment and legislative pressures to restrict immigration. From 1980 to 2010, the USA population increased 30%, to 310 million people. The 'White American' component of the national population increased by 9%, the 'African American' component increased 37%, 'Hispanic Americans' 175% and 'Asian Americans' 223%. By 2010, 50.5 million 'Hispanic Americans' comprised 16% of the total USA population. By 2010, 14.7 million 'Asian Americans' comprised 5% of the total USA population (Wintrob R, 2014). Between 2000 and 2010, the Hispanic American population grew by 30 percent; from 35.3 million in 2000 to 50.5 million in 2010. The increase in the Hispanic American population accounted for more than half of the 27.3 million increase in the total U.S. population (US Census Bureau reports;, 2010, 2011). The Asian American population grew 43 percent between 2000 and 2010; faster than any other racial/ethnic group. The Asian American population increased by 4.4 million; from 10.2 million in 2000 to 14.7 million in 2010.

The surge in ethnic diversity of immigrants over the past several decades portends even more dramatic demographic changes in the USA population– assuming that current immigration numbers continue through the next three decades. Demographic projections through 2050 are that the 'White American' component of the national population will decrease from >60% to <50% by 2050, the 'African American' component will increase from 13% to 15%, 'Hispanic Americans' will double, to >25% of the USA population, and 'Asian American' numbers will increase from 5% to 8%.

In the absence of a national consensus on immigration policy, and after nearly two decades of national government inaction and stalemate on immigration legislation, fear, resistance and hostility toward immigrants has been surging in USA. The issue has become more divisive still as anti-immigrant sentiment has been exploited in the lead-up to the 2016 Presidential election cycle.

Along with increased cultural diversity came the need to modify public health and medical service systems, education, employment, job training, housing and judicial services to better serve the more multicultural population. Concepts of 'cultural competence' and 'culturally sensitive clinical services' became widely accepted (Kohn R, Wintrob RM, Alarcon RD, 2009; Bhui K Warfa N, Edonya P, McKenzie K, Bhugra D, 2007). Service providers and administrators became more culturally diverse (Dein S, 2007; Ferguson J, Keller D, Haley H, Quirk M; 2003) Cultural diversity of staff started as a *'bottom up'* phenomenon; that is, people who worked somewhere in the health facility, but were not necessarily clinically trained, changing over time to medical and mental health clinicians who had some interest and experience in cultural issues related to health, and finally, involving the active participation of highly trained and experienced mental health clinicians, representing the *'top down'* integration of clinical staff.

Person-centered Care in Health and Mental Health; Looking to the Future

The fundamental premise of this presentation is that the steady increase in cultural diversity and multicultural societies throughout the world require that all clinicians who regularly encounter people in multicultural environments need to have the educational background and clinical experience to confidently provide culturally sensitive and individually tailored treatment appropriate for their needs. Consistent with this perspective, it should be a reasonable expectation that the administrative staff that supports clinicians, and clinicians themselves, will be increasingly culturally diverse in the decades ahead, better reflecting the demographic characteristics of the populations they serve (Cloninger CR, Zohar AH. Cloninger KM; 2010). This requires a broadening of perspective that starts with taking account of people's racial, ethnic and religious backgrounds, their family structure and function, their migration history, their language preferences and fluency, their community affiliations and their experiences with acculturation and acculturative stress (Kohn R, Wintrob RM, Alarcon, RD; 2015, in press).

Concerning family structure, function and dynamics, clinicians need to be familiar with the concepts of inter-generational communication, inter-generational differences in cultural adaptation and integration, the use of children as 'culture brokers' in immigrant families, and inter-generational conflict of values during the process of acculturation (Berry JW; 2003, Kohn R, Wintrob RM, Alarcon, RD; 2015, in press). Familiarity with these concepts will enable clinicians to more competently assess the impact that acculturative stress, experiences of cultural exclusion and discrimination have on the symptom presentation of individuals and families. It will improve rapport and enable them to better assess the coping abilities of individuals and families, as well as their responsiveness to and satisfaction with the clinical care that is offered to them (Group for the Advancement of Psychiatry, Committee on Cultural Psychiatry; 2002). Clinicians need to know that the process of acculturation affects communities as a whole, just as it does families and individuals; that both acculturation and adaptation to acculturative stress play out across several generations, that there may be very significant differences in intra-familial and inter-generational ability to cope with acculturative stress. In the larger societal context, clinicians need to be sensitive to the impact of socio-political currents that have a direct and powerful effect on national policy toward immigration and immigrants. National policies may vary considerably over time between the poles of hostility toward immigration, with fear and resentment of immigrants at the 'rejection' pole, to encouragement and support for both immigration and immigrants at the 'acceptance' pole. Changes in national sentiment can be unexpected and severe. Nations that had been characterized by an 'open door' policy toward immigration can change to feeling so fearful and overwhelmed by the pressures of surging numbers of immigrants and refugees that there is a clamor to wall off the borders and ghetto-ize all recent migrants.

Cultural Elements of the Relationship Between the Individual and the Clinician; Incorporating Cultural Formulation in Clinical Assessment

It is clear that differences in cultural characteristics between the individual, the family and the clinician can have profound effects on diagnosis, treatment adherence and satisfaction with the overall experience of care. Rapport is essential to this process, and is largely determined by the ease of communication between everyone involved, the establishment and maintenance of respectful social distance, empathic questioning and allowing individuals and families time to explain their presenting problems and their efforts to have tried to cope with the stressors they have experienced.

To accomplish this there has been a steady evolution in culturally informed techniques and procedures over the past two decades (De Jong J, Van Ommeren M, 2005; Group for the Advancement of Psychiatry, Committee on Cultural Psychiatry: 2002, Ton H, Lim RF; 2006).

The 'Outline for Cultural Formulation' was first included in DSM-IV and published in 1994 (American Psychiatric Association, Diagnostic and Statistical Manual of Mental Disorders, 1994). The purpose of Cultural Case Formulation was to provide a systematic review of the individual's and the family's cultural background, to identify the role of the cultural context in the expression and evaluation of medical and psychiatric dysfunction and symptoms, and to enhance the application of medical and psychiatric diagnostic criteria in culturally diverse, multicultural environments. The premise of clinicians conducting a culturally informed diagnostic formulation was that it would help clarify the extent to which cultural factors affect diagnosis and determine treatment plans. That in turn would help in identifying the likelihood of acceptance, and compliance with, recommended medical and psychiatric treatment. It would lead clinicians to explore with individuals and their families the likelihood of their involvement in simultaneous complementary, alternative, folk, indigenous, faith/spiritual or other healing procedures. Clinicians were urged to talk with patients and their families about their cultural identity, including their ethnic or cultural reference groups, their migration histories and their language preferences and fluency. They were urged to discuss the 'idioms of distress' through which their symptoms were expressed in relation to the norms of their cultural reference groups, and the perceived causes or 'explanatory models' they used or were influenced by. It was recommended that clinicians also explore cultural factors related to psychosocial environment and levels of functioning, cultural elements of the relationship with the clinician, and make an overall cultural assessment fir diagnosis and care.

However, the lack of inclusion of a specific set of questions on each of these topics proved to be a serious limitation to the widespread use of the Outline for Cultural Formulation.

Cultural Case Formulation in DSM-5; Inclusion of the 'Cultural Formulation Interview'

In an effort to address the limitations of the Outline for Cultural Formulation contained in DSM-4 and in its subsequent text revision (American Psychiatric Association, Diagnostic and Statistical Manual of Mental Disorders, 2000), the Cultural Psychiatry Working Group for DSM-5 developed the more structured 'Cultural Formulation Interview' that was incorporated in the DSM-5 (American Psychiatric Association, Diagnostic and Statistical Manual of Mental Disorders, 2013). The rationale, background and conceptual framework of the Cultural Formulation Interview have been elaborated in a separate volume (Lewis-Fenandez R, Aggarwal NK, Hinton L, Hinton DE, Kirmayer LJ; 2015).

The Cultural Formulation Interview explicitly recognizes cultural variation in symptom presentation. It recognizes cross-cultural and regional variation, as well as intra-cultural and intra-familial variation in symptom presentation and prevalence, and it recognizes and validates cultural assessment as a component of 'person-centered care' in medicine and in psychiatry (Mezzich JE; 2007) It enables clinicians to operationalize concepts inherent in cultural case formulation. Interview questions can be readily applied for use with family members and other informants, to provide socio-cultural context. Furthermore, it emphasizes collaborative, shared decision-making concerning diagnosis and treatment.

The Cultural Formulation Interview consists of four sections, comprising 16 questions. The sections of the interview, and the questions contained in each section are;

- *Cultural definition of the presenting problem*
  - Subject's definition/description of the problem/situation
  - Subject's description of problem to others in family, friends, community
  - Subject's description of most troubling aspects of problem
- *Cultural perceptions of cause, context and support available*
  - Subject's description of cause of presenting problem
  - Subject's description of cause according to family, friends and other community contacts
  - How subject's environment is helpful
  - How subject's environment is stressful
- *Role of cultural identity*
  - Description of key aspects of subject's background or identity
  - Effect of subject's background or identity on problem
  - Other concerns regarding subject's cultural identity
- *Cultural factors affecting coping and health seeking*
  - Methods subject has been using for self-coping
  - Methods and sources subject has used for coping in past
  - How subject's environment is helpful
  - Barriers subject has encountered to getting help for identified problem
- There are two additional sections. They are;

- *Current help-seeking practices and preferences*
  - Help subject has found most useful at this time
  - Other types of help suggested by family, friends and other community contacts
- *Misunderstandings in clinician-patient relationship*
  - Subject's concerns about this issue

– Subject's views about what can be done to get subject appropriate help Clinicians are also encouraged to use an outline of questions that are included in twelve 'Supplementary Modules' for more detailed exploration of issues related to explanatory model; level of functioning; social network; psychosocial stressors; spirituality, religion, and moral traditions; cultural identity; coping and help-seeking; patient–clinician relationship; school-age children and adolescents; older adults; immigrants and refugees; and caregivers.

In Conclusion: Cultural Psychiatry from a Global Perspective

Since the main thrust of this presentation has been to describe and emphasize the application of cultural perspectives to clinical assessment in medical and mental health care, it seems highly appropriate to end the presentation by outlining some of the global implications of this approach.

I have tried to place clinical assessment and clinical care in the context of intense contemporary stressors related to intra-national and international conflict that have directly contributed to the biggest wave of migration the world has witnessed in over fifty years. This in turn has generated unanticipated and massive numbers of migrants around the world, millions of them living under and trying to cope with severe stress and recurrent trauma, desperately seeking safety, acceptance and opportunity for a better life for themselves and their families.

As care providers and as concerned citizens of a turbulent world, we strive to alleviate misery and make life better for people to the extent we can contribute. Providing culturally sensitive, responsive and empathic treatment is our goal. Applying the concepts of cultural relativity, sensitive assessment and supportive treatment can be a direct benefit to the culturally diverse, multicultural populations we are committed to serve.

This perspective recognizes the human cost of psychiatric illness; the 'global burden of disease' and its functional impairment for individuals, families and communities (Global Burden of Disease Study Collaborators; 2013). It emphasizes 'the burden of social stigma' psychiatric illness imposes on individuals, families and communities, including the added burdens related to ethnic, racial and religious minority status and discrimination (Burnett-Zeiler I, Bohnert K, Illgen MA; 2013, Kohn R, Saxena S, Levav I, Saraceno B; 2004). It highlights the deleterious impact of both stigma and psychiatric illness on nations' growth and development. It emphasizes the integration of all psychiatric services with primary care, and related community services. It emphasizes cost effectiveness of treatment and the prevention of disability. It also highlights relationships between psychiatric illness and social disadvantage, discrimination and impaired accessto educational and occupational opportunity (Rodriguez-Seijas, Stohl M, Hasin DS, Eaton NR; 2015)

And finally, this approach recognizes the potential for the achievement of bi-national and bi-cultural identity as an outcome of adequately coping with acculturative stress in the 21st century (Schwartz SJ, Montgomery MJ, Briones E; 2006, Wintrob R; 2014).

References

American Psychiatric Association, Committee on Transcultural Psychiatry; Position Statement on the Delineation of Transcultural Psychiatry as a Specialized Field of Study. Amer J Psychiatry 1969, 126: 453–455.

American Psychiatric Association, Diagnostic and Statistical Manual of Mental Disorders, Fourth Edition. Washington, 1994.

American Psychiatric Association, Diagnostic and Statistical Manual of Mental Disorders, Fourth Edition Text Revision. Washington, 2000.

American Psychiatric Association, Diagnostic and Statistical Manual of Mental Disorders, Fifth Edition. Washington, 2013.

Berry JW: Conceptual approaches to acculturation. In: Chun KM, Organista PB, Marin G, eds. Acculturation; Advances in Theory, Measurement and Applied Research. Washington. American Psychological Association; 2003:17–37.

Bhui K Warfa N, Edonya P, McKenzie K, Bhugra D. Cultural competence in mental health care: a review of model evaluations. BMC Health Services Research 2007; 7:15.

Burnett-Zeiler I, Bohnert K, Illgen MA: Ethnic identity, acculturation and the prevalence of lifetime psychiatric disorders among black, Hispanic, and Asian adults in the U.S. J Psychiatr Res. 2013; 47:56.

Cloninger CR, Zohar AH. Cloninger KM; Promotion of Well-Being in Person-Centered Mental Health Care. Focus; 2010 8:165–179.

Dein S: ABC of mental Health: Mental health in a multiethnic society.

BMJ 2007, 315:473–479.

De Jong J, Van Ommeren M: Mental Health Services in a Multicultural Society: Interculturalization and its Quality Surveillance.

Transcultural Psychiatry 2005, 42;437–456.

Ferguson J, Keller D, Haley H, Quirk M: Developing Culturally Competent Community Faculty: A Model Program Academic Medicine 2003, 78;1221–8.

Global Burden of Disease Study 2013 Collaborators; Global Burden of Diseases, Injuries, and Risk Factors Study 2013. The Lancet 2013, 386: 743–800.

Group for the Advancement of Psychiatry, Committee on Cultural Psychiatry: Cultural Assessment in Clinical Psychiatry. Washington: American Psychiatric Publishing, 2002.

Kohn R, Saxena S, Levav I, Saraceno B: The treatment gap in mental health care. Bull World Health Organ. 2004; 82:858.

Kohn R, Wintrob RM, Alarcon, RD: Transcultural Psychiatry. In: Saddock, BJ, Saddock, VA and Ruiz,P, eds. Comprehensive Textbook of Psychiatry. Volume 9. Philadelphia; Lippincott Williams and Wilkins. 2009; 734–753.

Kohn R, Wintrob RM, Alarcon, RD: Transcultural Psychiatry. In: Saddock, BJ, Saddock, VA and Ruiz,P, eds. Comprehensive Textbook of Psychiatry. Volume 10. Philadelphia; Lippincott Williams and Wilkins. 2015; in press.

Lewis-Fenandez R, Aggarwal NK, Hinton L, Hinton DE, Kirmayer LJ: DSM-5 Handbook on the Cultural Formulation Interview. Washington, American Psychiatric Publishing; 2015.

Mezzich JE. Psychiatry for the Person: articulating medicine's science and humanism. World Psychiatry. 2007, 6: 65–67.

Rodriguez-Seijas, Stohl M, Hasin DS, Eaton NR: Transdiagnostic factors and mediation of the relationship between perceived racial discrimination and mental disorders. JAMA Psychiatry. 2015 [Epub ahead of print].

Schwartz SJ, Montgomery MJ, Briones E. The role of identity in acculturation among immigrant people: Theoretical propositions, empirical questions, and applied recommendations. Human Development; 2006. 49, 1–30.

Ton H, Lim RF: The assessment of culturally diverse individuals. In: Lim RF, ed. Clinical Manual of Cultural Psychiatry. Washington. American Psychiatric Publishing; 2006: 3–31.

United Nations High Commission for Refugees: Annual Global Trends Report. Geneva, 2014.

United Nations High Commission for Refugees: Annual Global Trends Report. Geneva, 2015.

United States Census Bureau report. Washington. 2010

United States Census Bureau report. Washington. 2011

Wintrob R. The Scope and Influence of Cultural Psychiatry in a Turbulent World. Paper presented at the 8th Annual DTPPP Conference, Vienna; Sep 2014.

Short CV

Dr. Ronald M Wintrob MD
Psychiatrist
Blackstone
345 Blackstone Blvd
Providence, RI 02906

’I need a friend with who I may talk’ – qualitative survey

Ibrahim Özkan, Julia Vogel

The United Nations High Commissioner for Refugees declared at a conference on the Syrian Refugee Situation 2014 in Berlin:

‘First of all, there is a need for much stronger commitment to burden-sharing by other countries, allowing Syrian refugees to find protection beyond the immediate neighbouring region. This can be done through resettlement, humanitarian admission schemes, simplified family reunification or more flexible visa regulations.’ **1**

The political and social intercourse with traumatized refugees is an intensive discussed topic in the German society, due to the daily increasing stream of refugees. In reference to the statement of the United Nations High Commissioner for Refugees is a stronger commitment by the European community essential. In the conducted survey supported by the Network for Traumatized Refugees (NTFN) in 2012 was the first objective target to analyse the care situation for traumatized refugees in Lower Saxony. The current article contains the core results of the qualitative survey and a developed demand catalogue based on the conducted interviews. A case example of the interview Mr. L. outlines the key dynamics which determine the care situation of traumatized refugee in Lower Saxony. However, before the framework conditions, results and demand catalogue are represented, a brief overview of asylum trends is provided for the year 2014.

Asylum Trends 2014

The Asylum Trends 2014 published by the UNHCR summarizes individual asylum claims submitted in Europe during 2014. The report presents a registration of 173,100 new asylum application in Germany. Thus, Germany continues to be the largest single recipient of new asylum claims among the group of industrialized countries, i.e. on average, every fifth application in the 44 industrialized countries was obtained by Germany. **2** In 2014, international protection was requested by the highest number of people from the Syrian Arab Republic, Serbia and Kosovo, Eritrea, Afghanistan as well as Albania. The reason for the sharp increase in the number of asylum-seekers registered among industrialised countries is a combination of armed conflict, deterioration of security or humanitarian situation and human rights. A high increase of asylum applicants can be observed within the last five years.

As the UN High Commissioner for refugees points out:

'Today, the surge in armed conflicts around the world presents us with similar challenges. Our response has to be just as generous now as it was then – providing access to asylum, resettlement opportunities and other forms of protection for the people fleeing these terrible conflicts.'

Context and target of the qualitative survey

On this account, the NTFN (Network for Traumatized Refugees in Lower Saxony) and the Leibniz University Hannover developed the idea to conduct a survey with the pivotal request to expose the supply situation of traumatized refugees. The designated target of the qualitative survey has been an exploitation of the care situation of traumatized refugees in the federate state Lower Saxony. Moreover, in comparison to further federate states such as Berlin, Bremen or North Rhine-Westphalia, Lower Saxony is one of the few federate states which does not possess a region wide care.

Thus, 29 persons based on the research method Grounded Theory (GMT) by Glaser and Strauss as well as guided interviews construction by Helfferich from seven different occupational groups (lawyers, doctors, psychotherapists, psychiatrists, social workers, skilled workers in public institutions, interpreters) have been interviewed as well as experts, volunteers and refugees. **3, 4, 5** The reason for applying GMT was the claim to detect the supply situation of traumatized refugees out of various perspective to point out groups of players as well as collect demands of different working groups. These demands were compiled to an encompassing catalogue. This demand catalogue has been developed by the research methods of open and selected coding through code families in applying the research program Atlas.ti. Based on the results of the open and selective coding social process operations could be revealed and described, but a new middle-range theory complaint with the target of Glaser and Strauss was not generated. Therefore, conducted study has to be understood as a first glance on the care situation of traumatized refugees in Lower Saxony.

The interviewees cooperate actively with the NTFN and endorse traumatized refugees within their daily field of work. Since 2014 the NTFN established a crisis intervention center for traumatized refugees in Hannover. The KIZ is funded by the government of Lower Saxony and the European Fund for Refugees. In 2014, the employees of the KIZ supervised 414 cases and the most frequent country of origin like Syria, Sudan and Eritrea. **6** The foundation of the KIZ has been a long-awaited goal of the NTFN and a principal object of the conducted study.

The importance of the conducted survey is due to the fact that refugees are exposed to a considerably increased vulnerability during the migration process **7** and within the clinical context Freyberger & Widder pointed out a high number of stressors in the course of the asylum procedure, e.g. loneliness, unemployment and uncertainty according to permit of residence. These stressors influence the posttraumatic stress disorder (PTSB) and may also possess reinforcing effects. **8, 9** The subjective fear of deportation correlates verifiable with the symptom severity, $r = .67$. Consequently, the thesis could be confirmed that the symptom severity of a PTSB is coherent with an uncertain residence status. **10** Further on, Lindert, Brähler, Wittig, Mieleck & Priebe describe a lack of reliable data about the health status of migrants and especially refugees in Germany. **11** Such a lack of data has become as well apparent during the theoretical research process of health data in Lower Saxony for the present survey. On this account, an investigation of the care situation of Lower Saxony was judicious and the core results of the survey refer firstly, to ascertained centrifugal, obstructing and integrative dynamics and these secondly, determine the development of a demand catalogue.

The influence of centrifugal, obstructing and integrative dynamics on the supply situation

For the analysis of the care situation the research model of Ursula Brucks and Wulf-Bodo Wahls has been utilized as the basis for the current survey. **12** The research model has been developed within the framework of a survey about the health and living conditions of immigrants in four federate states by the Robert-Koch-Institute. Therefore, the analysis of the empirical data is premised on the research model. The model contains a particular investigation of obstacles and impediments in the health care system. Brucks und Wahls examined social dynamics and defined three different types of influencing factors: centrifugal, obstructing and integrative dynamics. Centrifugal dynamics induce negative effects, are bonded to structural conditions and require conflicts consistently. Obstructing dynamics do not generate ultimate negative effects, but the retardation of a professional treatment will be ensued. Obstructing dynamics might be narrowed down through counselling strategies and qualification measures of institutions. Integrative dynamics are accountable for the creation of counselling strategies and ascertain unconfined access to the health care system. The aspirations of integrative dynamics are emancipated participation in the health care system and an enhancement of political strategies to guarantee medical as well as social care for aggrieved groups.

The results of the conducted survey demonstrated that centrifugal dynamics exist in the shape of the right of residence, obsolescent working process in governmental institutions, high costs to retain a lawyer or a psychological expert assessment which are indispensable while a direct action access in court. Additionally, the clarification of costs, decision-finding in reference to an approval of trauma or PTBS by the court as well as the temporary accommodation are destabilizing the symptoms. Moreover, the uncertainty and non-transparency on the part of governmental institutions and concerning the German bill might lead to reinforcement of the symptoms.

Furthermore, Lower Saxony is an area state which implies a reasonable care in the cities and a severe undercare in the rural areas. A psychotherapist who works in the locality of Lüneburg reported about the lack of therpeutic capacity and the only possibility for a comprehensive treatment is an inpatient admission. Outpatient-working therapist are not able or overchallenged to treat traumatized refugees.

Further on, the interviewed occupational groups described obstructing dynamics in applying for the absorption of costs of therapy positions, fares and interpreters by governmental institutions. Auxiliary barriers of the care situation are the conditions of the German social welfare Law for asylum seekers and the costs of medical estimates. Psychiatrists and (medical) psychotherapists delineate that the issue of medical estimates takes up a lot of time and is not affordable for registered psychiatrists and psychotherapists. Particularly, in rural areas the care situation of traumatised refugees has been perceived as limited and unsustainable by the interviewed occupational groups based on the skilled worker shortage and lack of expert knowledge.

"(...) Lower Saxony is an area state. This is of course, the biggest problem, if I see, where people have been transferred, where I attempted in Ochte, that is the administrative district of Nienburg, in the direction to Bremen or in Loccum-Rehberg, to receive a point of contact to a migration or refugee advice centre. There is nothing!" (translated quotation of interview 3, Line 1445–1451). **13**

The shortage of knowledge and a poor sensitization on the subject of trauma within the governmental institutions (courts, foreigners' registration office, Federal Office for Migration and Refugees) exacerbate the professional care and treatment of traumatized refugees. Without the support of healthcare professionals in this crisis situation, the cluster of symptoms would not be bearable by PTBS or trauma patients.

For this very reason, an intensive network of cooperation between NGOs, public institutions and players of various occupational groups is imperative to the reduction of barriers within the care situation. Integrative dynamics are the collaborative work between NGOs like the NTFN, Treatment Centers for Torture Victims (e.g. Refugio, XENION), the Refugee Council of Lower Saxony, church-based institution and registered associations as the Ethno-Medical Centre. These different facilities are toeholds between governmental institutions and traumatized refugees. They render legal consultation, assist in the search for therapy or assessments and financial support for example in case of interpreter costs or travel costs. The results pointed out that the main targets of these associations are a cultural opening of public and governmental institutions, professional groups and the society, i.e. a seizure of possibilities for participation to organize a care situation for traumatized refugees (cp. Vogel 2012: 109). Further, based on the network of the associations different occupational groups started to collaborate with each other and developed a strong help structure to surmount peripheral isolation and to ensure a general supply.

The analysis of the interviews indicated different demand on the behalf of the occupational groups. These demands were identified through the selective coding and compiled in a demand catalogue.

Development of a Demand catalogue by the generated data

The demands refer to on a reduction of centrifugal dynamics which are oriented on the structural conditions in Lower Saxony (reducing differences between the rural and urban areas), juridical determining factors and regular practices of public institutions. The superior target of the occupation groups is a nationwide care of traumatized refugees in the social, public and medical sector. Hence, it is regarded to eliminate social disparity between the peripheral rural and central urban position. Consequently, the occupational groups claim an expansion of the care and treatment situation within the local authority. An additional change of desire is based on the juridical determining factors in Germany, i.e. a demand on an abolition of the German social welfare Law for asylum seekers as well as independent legal regulation of the refugee law. The overriding objective is an acceleration to access societal sub-areas such as the employment market, education opportunities in the course of the asylum procedure and a faster approval of educational qualifications. Thus, accessing the health, legal, education and social system has to be facilitated to enable a comprehensive support of traumatized refugees.

In compliance with the statements of the occupational groups, an acceleration of participation within the German society is badly needed, for example a clarification of the functional responsibility of benefactors and amendments of the condition of admission. On this account, the access to respective societal sections (health care, judicial and social system) has to be simplified with the objective of enabling inclusion of traumatized refugees.

Obstructing dynamics might be restricted through educational work and broadening of the sensibility of the disease pattern PTBS and trauma. The occupation groups emphasized that an understanding of the symptoms has to be developed in every social section, because of the specific vulnerability of traumatized refugees. The reduction of obstructing dynamics might be also limited by means of a shift within the current health care trend. Therefore, the interviewees require an encompassing care of traumatized refugees, a fast psychological and social treatment, native language therapists, (psychic) supervision of each occupational group and appreciation of personal borders. These demands are addressed to the health care system and functional responsibility of the benefactors (public health office, social welfare office, public health fund). Ultimately, bureaucratic *procedures* and concessions of therapies or cost absorption have to be accelerated, in order to prevent a destabilization of traumatized refugees. Consequently, the development as well as provision of a comprehensive care and therapy concept in the commune is claimed to surmount social disparity and foster inclusive processes for traumatized refugees.

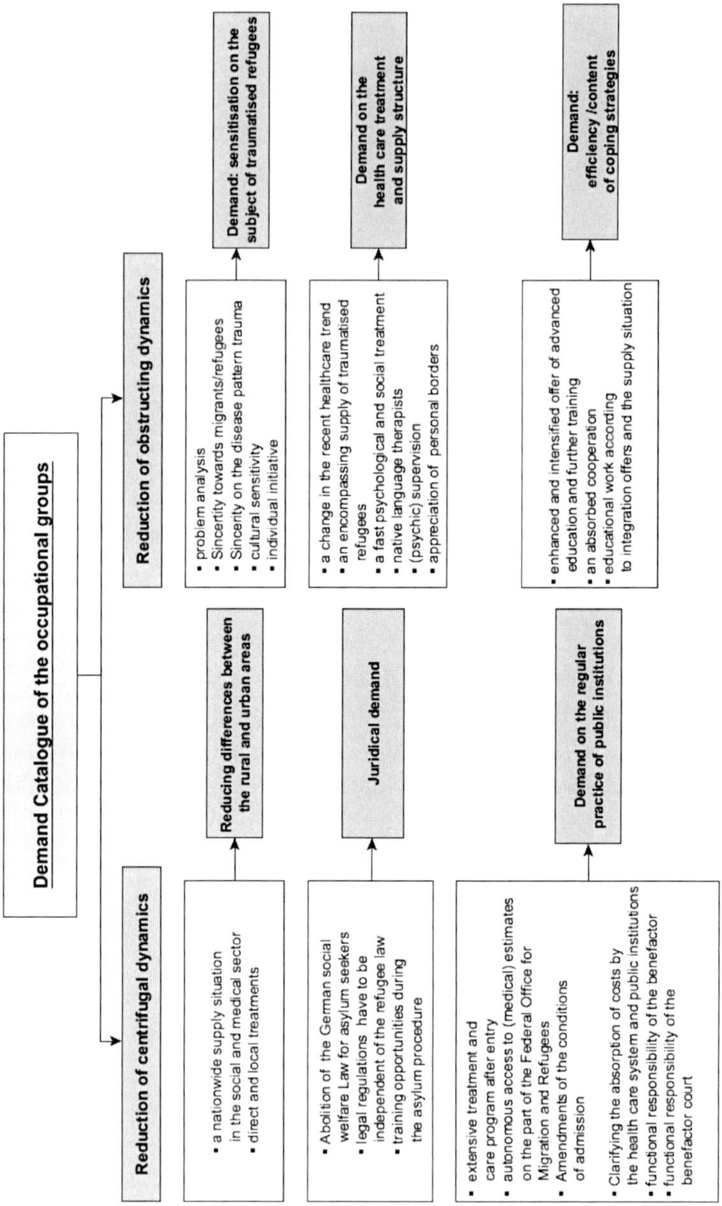
Demand Catalogue of the occupational groups
Reduction of centrifugal dynamics
Reduction of obstructing dynamics
▪ a nationwide supply situation in the social and medical sector
▪ direct and local treatments
Reducing differences between the rural and urban areas
▪ Abolition of the German social welfare Law for asylum seekers
▪ legal regulations have to be independent of the refugee law
▪ training opportunities during the asylum procedure
Juridical demand
▪ extensive treatment and care program after entry
▪ autonomous access to (medical) estimates on the part of the Federal Office for Migration and Refugees
▪ Amendments of the conditions of admission
▪ Clarifying the absorption of costs by the health care system and public institutions
▪ functional responsibility of the benefactor
▪ functional responsibility of the benefactor court
Demand on the regular practice of public institutions
▪ problem analysis
▪ Sincertity towards migrants/refugees
▪ Sincerity on the disease pattern trauma
▪ cultural sensitivity
▪ individual initiative
Demand: sensitisation on the subject of traumatised refugees
▪ a change in the recent healthcare trend
▪ an encompassing supply of traumatised refugees
▪ a fast psychological and social treatment
▪ native language therapists
▪ (psychic) supervision
▪ appreciation of personal borders
Demand on the health care treatment and supply structure
▪ enhanced and intensified offer of advanced education and further training
▪ an absorbed cooperation
▪ educational work according to integration offers and the supply situation
Demand: efficiency /content of coping strategies

3. Case study of a refugee in Lower Saxony- an illustration of integrative dynamics

'I do not need clothes, a television, a carpet or bed; I need a friend with whom I may talk. I am alone here since four months. Whatever happened in Iran, I was totally under stress, and now I need somebody who get in touch with me.' (translated quotation of interview 21, Mr. L., Line 7933–7946)

The interviewee Mr. L. described his first impressions after the arrival in Germany. In terms of the quotation, during his first four months, Mr. L. could not speak the language, he had no work just a single bed with a number and he was searching a friend. A person who listens to his current problems and experiences which he made in his state of origin. Therefore, he went to the social welfare work 'Diakonie' and he did not ask for furniture, food or money, he just needed a person who talk to. The employees of the 'Diakonie' developed various solutions to integrate Mr. L. in the community and become an active part in the church congregation.

In the course of the first four months, Mr. L. mentioned a lot of difficulties in relation to registration, allocation in the communities, and the lack of support on the part of government agencies. Also, insufficient language skills, a lack of knowledge regarding the German health care system as well as German jurisdiction and restrained information policy were major obstacles within the integration process. These hurdles ascribe the obstructing dynamics in Lower Saxony.

Nevertheless, through the employees of the Diakonie, Mr. L. became acquainted with the NTFN because he was searching for juridical support of his asylum procedure and to receive a therapy place. The NTFN appealed to the Asklepios Hosptial in Göttingen and Mr. L. obtained a therapy place. Further on, even if Mr. Ls. asylum application was denied repeatedly for the fourth time, the NFTN organized juridical support and ascertain every reasonable practical step to encourage Mr. L. This delineates decisively the imperative necessity of integrative dynamics. The psychotherapists (of the Asklepios Hosptial in Göttingen) Özkan and Belz postulate a close network with therapists, institutions and organizations to improve the care situation for traumatized refugees:

'For a better care of traumatized patients with a history of migration a professional networking with psychotherapist as well as interested colleagues have to be promote' (comp. Özkan, Belz 2013: 216).

With the goal to treat traumatized patients in the best possible way Dr. Özkan developed the 'Göttinger Concept' which can be seen as pioneer in treatment of traumatized patients. The concept is combination of therapeutic methods (EMDR, TRUST, CIPBS, PITT and DBT), **14** bilingual therapy, inclusion of interpreters, supervision and the development of new therapeutic materials without a language-based approach. The concept targets to prevent frustration and helplessness induced by language barriers and insufficient language skills on the behalf of the patients. Thus, the main pillars of the concept regard cultural diversity, ensuring of stability and elaboration of coping strategies. **15**

Mr. L. would have not obtained any support neither juridical nor therapeutic without the strong network structure between the Diakonie, NTFN and Asklepios Hospital. Consequently, Integrative dynamics created by different key players are indispensable and required to provide traumatized refugees with various dimensions of support and reduce in the same way centrifugal as well as obstructing dynamics. In end, Mr. L. pictured quite impressively that through the network structure he was not any longer a number in a system, he became a person.

The positive proof of centrifugal, obstructing and integrative dynamics in Lower Saxony was the key target of the qualitative survey. The existence of three operating different dynamics lead to the development of a demand catalogue based on the statements of seven interview groups. As the pivotal points of the demand catalogue sharply illustrate, is an urgently required reduction of centrifugal and obstructing dynamics. Projects of the NTFN or the Göttinger Concepts are effective countermeasures, nevertheless, further implementations are required for a comprehensive supply of traumatized refugees in area state Lower Saxony

References

1 United Nation High Commissioner for Refugees UNHCR (2014): Remarks by António Guterres, United Nations High Commissioner for Refugees. Conference on the Syrian Refugee Situation – Supporting Stability in the Region. Berlin, 28 October 2014. Available at: http://www.unhcr.org/544fb4189.html [19.07.2015].

2 United Nation High Commissioner for Refugees UNHCR (2015): Asylum Trends 2014, Levels and Trends in Industrialized Countries. Geneva.

3 Helfferich, C. (2011): Die Qualität qualitativer Daten. Manual für die Durchführung qualitativer Interviews. In: Qualität qualitativer Daten.

4 Flick, U. (2011): Triangulation. Eine Einführung. 3. Aufl. Wiesbaden: VS Verlag für Sozialwissenschaften (Qualitative Sozialforschung, 12).

5 Glaser, B.-G.; Strauss, A. L. (2005): Grounded theory. Strategien qualitativer Forschung. 2., korrigierte Aufl. Bern: Huber (Gesundheitswissenschaften: Methoden).

6 Netzwerk für traumatisierte Flüchtlinge in der Niedersachsen e.V. (2014): Sachbericht 2014. Available at: http://www.ntfn.de/wp-content/uploads/2013/06/PSZ-Bericht-13--14.pdf [19.07.2015].

7 Silove, D., Sinnerbrink, I., Field, A., Manicavasagar, V., Steel, Z. (1997): Anxiety, depression and PTSD in asylum seekers: associations with pre-migration trauma and post-migration stressors. In: The British Journal of Psychiatry, H. 170, 351–357.

8 Freyberger, H.- J., Widder, B. (2010): Begutachtung von Traumatisierungen. In: Psychotherapeut, H. 55, 401–408.

9 Odenwald, M., Schmitt, T., Neuner, F., Ruf, M., Schauer, M. (2006): Aussageverhalten von traumatisierten Flüchtlingen. Eine Untersuchung zum Vorbringen des eigenen Verfolgungsschicksals im Rahmen des Asylverfahrens. In: Zeitschrift für Politische Psychologie, H. 14 (1–2), 225–253.

10 Gerlach, C., Pietrowsky, R. (2012): Trauma und Aufenthaltsstatus. Einfluss eines unsicheren Aufenthaltsstatus auf die Traumasymptomatik bei Flüchtlingen. In: Verhaltenstherapie & Verhaltensmedizin, H. 33 (1), 5–19.

11 Lindert, J., Brähler, E., Wittig, U., Mielck, A., Priebe, S. (2008): Depressivität, Angst und posttraumatische Belastungsstörung bei Arbeitsmigranten, Asylbewerbern und Flüchtlingen. Systematische Übersichtsarbeit zu Originalstudien. In: Psychother Psych Med, H. 58, 109–122.

12 Brucks, U., Wahl, W.-B. (2003): Über-, Unter-, Fehlversorgung? Bedarfslücken und Strukturprobleme in der ambulanten Gesundheitsversorgung von Migrantinnen und Migranten. In: Borde, T., David, M. (Hrsg.) Gut versorgt? Migrantinnen und Migranten im Gesundheits- und Sozialwesen. Frankfurt am Main: Mabuse-Verlag.

13 Vogel, Julia (2012): Eine qualitative Untersuchung der Versorgungsstrukturen traumatisierter Flüchtlinge im Bundesland Niedersachsen (Master Thesis). Leibniz Universität Hanover (unpublished).

14 Özkan, I., Belz, M. (2013): Ressourcenorientierte traumazentrierte Behandlung von Migranten. In: Feldmann, R-E,. Jr., Seidler, G. (Hrsg.), Traum(a) Migration. Aktuelle Konzepte zur Therapie traumatisierter Flüchtlinge und Folteropfer. Gießen: Psychosozial-Verlag.

15 Özkan, I., Belz, M. (2010): Behandlungskonzepte für Menschen mit Migrationshintergrund. In: Heise, T., Golsabahi, S. (Hrsg.), Mit Leib und Seele ankommen. 09. – 11. Dezember 2010, Ärztekammer Nordrhein, Düsseldorf. Berlin: VWB, Verl. für Wiss. und Bildung (Kongress des Dachverbands der Transkulturellen Psychiatrie, Psychotherapie und Psychosomatik im Deutschsprachigen Raum e.V.(DTPPP), 4).

Short CV

Ibrahim Özkan
E-mail: i.oezkan@asklepios.com
Adress: Asklepios Fachklinikum Göttingen, Rosdorfer Weg 70, 37081 Göttingen
Phone: +49–551+402–1650

Graduated psychologist and certified psychological psychotherapist, works as main employment in the out-patient department of the psychiatric hospital “Asklepios Fachklinikum Göttingen “, Rosdorfer Weg 70, 37081 Göttingen, Germany. Here he is the superviser of the clinical expert-team for culture, migration and mental illness. He works as medical psychologist, is scientific employee at the departement for social science and he has a teaching assignment at the center for key-competences at the art departement of the Georg-Augusta-University of Göttingen. As coach, docent, supervisor and consultant of different institutions concerning his key subjects, he obtained profound experiences over many years. Core subjects are a.o. migration, migration and mental health, psychotrauma, refugees, intercultural work in mental healthcare, practice management and psycho-oncology.

Therapeutical core subjects:

- qualified traumatherapy (DeGPT), qualified EMDR, DBT, qualified psycho-oncology, TRUST, CIPBS
- expert consultant on the topic PTSD and migration

On this subjects he accomplished different national and international publications, lectures, symposia and workshops. Besides, he is active member of the AIKUD, an istitution for universal and intercutural didactics, member of the GTP, a society for turkish speaking psychotherapy and psychosocial consulting, joint founder and board member of the DTPPP, the confederation of transcultural psychiatry and psychosomatics of german speaking countries, board member at the european society of integration in medical healthcare, consultant and scientific attendant of different european projects.

Julia Vogel

B.A. Social Sciences, Postgraduate Training to Traumata-Advisor, is a current Master student in the area of Atlantic Studies at the Leibniz University Hannover. She has been working as research assistant in the Asia-Pacific Center for the Responsibility to Protect at University of Queensland (Brisbane, Australia) and currently, possesses a position as a student assistant in the HIS company (Higher Education Information System). Furthermore, she holds a leading position within the UNICEF Working Group in Hannover.

RETREAT – Ressource Establishing Trauma Relief Elaboration And Treatment

Ibrahim Özkan, Maria Belz

Immigration rates in Germany have steadily increased since 2006 (Federal Office for Migration and Refugees, 2015). In the last years, the percentage of immigrants seeking asylum (2013: + 83,2%), as well as those for humanitarian reasons (2013: + 44,9%) has increased dramatically in Germany. Within this population, there is a high need for psychotherapeutic and psychiatric care. Their traumatic experiences vary from persecution and torture in their home countries, violence on the way to the host country up to domestic violence (Özkan, 2013). These traumatic experiences, coupled with the acculturative stress that even comes with regular migration and is extended by asylum seekers, can increase the risk for psychological crisis, particularly in this population (e.g. Brucks, 2004).

In a representative survey at 171 psychiatric outpatients' departments in Germany, 32,5% of the interviewed patients had an immigration background (Schouler-Ocak, Bretz, Hauth, Heredia Montesinos et al., 2010). Nevertheless, migrants are a patient group, which uses the psychological and psychiatric care system below average, although there is a higher risk for psychological disorders in this population (National psychotherapeutic association, 2010). The insufficient supply to treatment offers and lack of information for this patient group about the services have been identified as influencing factors, among others.

If a patient who has experienced the trauma cited above has managed to overcome the obstacles that come with accessing adequate treatment in Germany, they find another obstacle in managing to communicate effectively with their therapist (Özkan & Belz, 2014). Learning German as a migrant can be difficult for many. First, the demands of the living environment and immediate changes requiring an adaptive capacity and experiences of foreignness may constitute additional possible stress factors, impeding the learning of a foreign language (Özkan & Belz, 2014). Second, on the structural-political level, there is hardly any support for language learning. For example, there is no support for reimbursement for German courses for refugees who are still in the asylum procedures.

The language-barrier has been identified as one of the main reasons for the below-average utilization of psychotherapy (National psychotherapeutic association, 2010) and the difficulties for integrating migrants into the standard supply system (Özkan & Belz, 2013). Therefore, this element has to be urgently altered to improve the general situation for patients with migration background.

Vast evidence shows that "the lower the German-abilities, the higher the dissatisfaction with the treatment, the therapeutic offers and the results" (p. 279, Bermejo, Berger, Kriston et al., 2009). Therefore, the outcome seems to be less important than a high-qualitative way of understanding.

There are experimental ways in which therapists and organizations are trying to mitigate the obstacles migrants face while trying to adapt in Germany and access adequate psychological treatment. Amongst them are: treatment in their native language, use of translators in the therapy, use of language-reduced psychotherapeutic methods, and use of culturally sensitive treatment concepts.

Treatment in mother tongue should be amplified, so that at least a verbal understanding between therapist and patient can be guaranteed (National psychotherapeutic association, 2010). By appreciating the native language, the patient's satisfaction as well as the compliance could be improved (Özkan & Belz, 2013). Unfortunately, emerging problems, such as the accessibility to mother tongued therapists in poorly structured areas are difficult to surmount.

Another possible way of overcoming the language-barrier is to work with translators. However, in practice the collaboration often fails because of deficient qualification or other structural problems such as insufficient financing (Wolf & Özkan, 2012) or because patients feel uncomfortable about a third person's presence during the therapeutic treatment.

Due to the mentioned difficulties regarding the collaboration with translators and the work with mother tongued therapists, it is crucial for an appropriate treatment, to develop language-reduced psychotherapeutic methods, forming a part of culture-sensitive treatment concepts.

In the following, language-reduced methods for psychotherapeutic settings are introduced (RETREAT – Ressource Establishing Trauma Relief Elaboration And Treatment) (Özkan & Belz, 2013). The methods derive from the salutogenetic approach (Antonovsky, 1996) and are embedded in a broader trauma therapeutic concept. Subsequently the concept for a trauma-stabilisation-group for patients with migration background as a possible setting for language-reduced intervention is presented. Afterwards the libra, the trauma cubes and the chain reaction as three principal language-reduced methods will be explained in detail.

The salutogenetic approach in language-reduced methods and trauma-therapy

The language-reduced methods presented in the following paper aim to empower the patients in order to give them the resources to revert in burdening situations. Furthermore, they reinforce protective factors in accordance with the sense of coherence (SOC) in Antonovskys salutogenic approach (Antonovsky, 1996). Antonovsky emphasizes the aspects of (1) manageability, in our setting understood in the literal sense of "palpable with the hand", (2) meaningfulness and (3) comprehensibility.

Furthermore, the language-reduced methods developed at the Asklepios Fachklinikum Göttingen (specialized psychiatric clinic) have been generated specifically considering trauma-therapy, in which the three factors of sense of coherence (SOC) are very important as well:

(1) Manageability: If a traumatic experience has been subject of discussion in the therapeutic session, or the patient experiences intrusions or flashbacks during the session, it may be quite destabilizing, especially if the burdening situation hasn't been completely processed by the patient and taken home as an emotional load. Methods, which work with the traumatic

incidents visually, tangibly and in an exterior way have the great advantage, that patients can 'leave the burden' behind when they go home, leaving the subjective safety within the therapeutic setting.

(2) Meaningfulness: The extent to which a patient can discover meaning in the treatment or the structure of it as meaningful and significant experience (emotional representation) by engaging the structure and the sociocultural and traditional background of the patient.

(3) Comprehensibility: By using visual symbols and metaphors patients are better able to understand the content and aim of therapeutic interventions. Because of that also therapy taking place in mother tongue should use language-reduced methods as good complement taking in account that patients suffering of a stress disorder have less capacity reprocessing what is said.

The treatment of traumatized patients requires load capacity and a high ability of empathy from the therapist, as well as a high level of expertise (Teegen, 2000).

Therefore only experienced therapists, who are also able to handle dissociative states, a symptom shown often by traumatized patients (Teegen, 2000), as well as states of emergency in general, should use the RETREAT-methods presented in this paper.

It is recommended to apply the language-reduced methods after having developed a therapist-patient relationship first. A basic stabilisation should have been established as well.

The usage of RETREAT-methods has to be embedded into an overall treatment plan of trauma-centered psychotherapy: First of all, psychological assessments are conducted with the patient (e.g. with the IES, the BDI, the SCL-90-R, the QOL5, the ETI, etc.). After the diagnostic process, stabilisation is the first goal to attain in the therapy – either in group- or single-settings. When a basic stabilisation is achieved, therapist and patient begin to work with the traumatic experiences – if necessary, language-reduced methods can be used.

Traumasynthesis, the capacity to bear and to experience holistically the affect, the body sensations as well as other perceptual aspects of the traumatic situations (Sachsse, Schröder & Vogel, 2004), takes place by applying other confrontational procedures such as EMDR (Shapiro & Maxfield, 2002), CIPBS etc.

Trauma-Stabilisation-Group for Patients with migration background

Mendelsohn, Zachary and Harney (2007) have shown that the social aspects of group therapy counteract the isolating effect of interpersonal trauma, particularly for patients with posttraumatic stress disorder (PTSD). A general effectiveness of groups in psychotherapeutic care has been proven (Leszcz, 2004) and analysed (Agronin, 2009). It is for this reason that a trauma-stabilisation-group forms part of the "Göttingen treatment concept" for people with migration background (Özkan & Belz, 2013).

In this group-context it is as important to create a comfortable and confidential atmosphere (Hüther, 2004) in which patient and therapist find a way to communicate, as it is in single-setting.

An identified obstacle in the daily clinical practice is the lacking language-abilities of patients with migration background. This hinders the integration of these patients into therapeutic group-supply (Özkan, Belz, & Oktay, 2012).

Because of structural obstacles (such as many patients with different cultural backgrounds and mother languages), native-language group therapy is often difficult to implement in the daily practice. Language-reduced methods are therefore crucial and efficient for a group treatment for patients with migration background.

The trauma-stabilisation-group at the psychiatric outpatients' department (PIA) of the Asklepios Fachklinikum Göttingen focuses on a resources-orientated and language-reduced therapy. In this way, the therapist is aware of the benefits of speaking slowly and of using simple words, and is always mindful for utilizing gestures and symbols to illustrate of what is said. The usage of pictograms, symbols, items, posters and other visual tools provides a better environment for the patient's understanding, and further facilitates the process of learning coping-strategies. Therefore, the treatment-methods are transmitted in a tangible way.

The purpose of group therapy focuses on psychoeducation, the promotion of personal resources, as well as the learning of stabilisation-techniques, since these aspects are elementary for coping with psychological disorders, such as PTSD.

In this group-setting the patients elaborate individual strategies that will help them to deal with potentially triggering situations, such as how to deal with flashbacks by identifying potential triggers or learning how to reduce avoidance (Özkan & Belz, 2013).

Psychoeducation: The Libra

Psychoeducation has been proven to play a very important role for coping with psychological disorders (Liedl, Schäfer & Knaevelsrud, 2013). Its aim "to strengthen the patient's autonomy and promote their resources" (p. 1) is achieved by informing the patients in the clearest way about their disorder and dysfunctional automatisms.

The language-reduced method "Libra" illustrates and non-verbally explains Lazarus' and Folkman's transactional model of stress and coping (1984). With this Libra, there is a way of visualizing the imbalance between personal resources and burdens. This method can be applied in group-settings as well as in single-settings.

Required material:

1. A libra;
2. Black and white stones (e.g.);
3. A permanent marker and self-adhesive notepads, if necessary.

In a language-reduced, resources-orientated group-setting this method is useful to give a tangible and understandable introduction to the aims and reasons for the group work.

The therapist explains in a simple way that the patients are participating in the group- or single-therapy, because they have experienced traumatic, burdening situations and suffer psychological strain, which are illustrated by the black stones. They further explain that therapy won't be able to make this undone or disappear, while physically demonstrating this point by putting one or various black stones into one of the scale-pans.

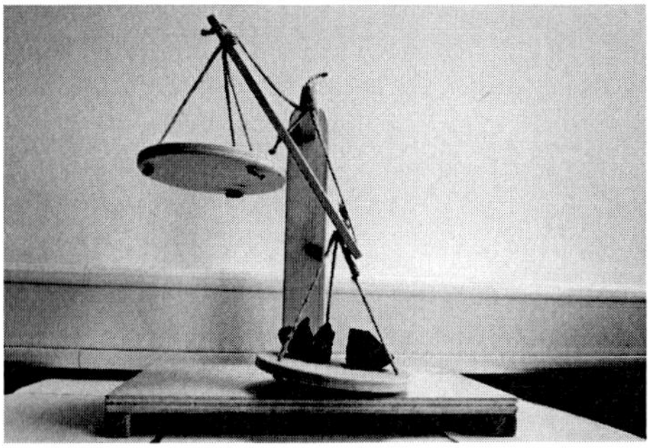

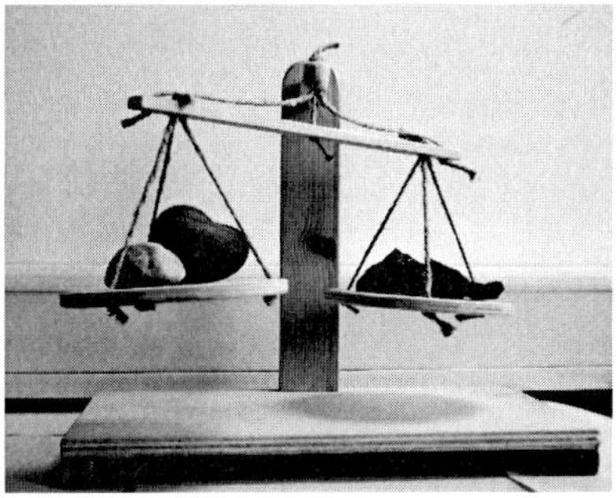

Together with the patient or the group, personal burdens are identified, either verbally, written on notepads or painted on paper and put on the stones.

With these actions, the libra is used to demonstrate that the burden is imbalanced, with the stones' weight on one pan, while not having any counterbalance on the other side.

In the next step of the therapy session, it is important to clarify that therapy (either in group or one-to-one) can help patients in finding ways to alleviate the weight of their negative experiences, and its effects in their daily lives.

These 'positive' weights, represented by the white stones used here, portray the personal resources patients are coached in identifying and adopting in their lives.

These resources can be activities or anything, that 'make one feel better', and by using them, can reduce the current stress-load (which has been illustrated by the balancing effect on the libra). For patients with migration background it is helpful to point out that resources may also be activities, things or thoughts they know from their home-countries, yet have not been utilizing them being outside of their native homes (Belz & Özkan, 2013).

With this physical representation of stress with therapy tools, patients can understand more easily in a speech-reduced way and experience the function of resources: while they are not able to make the burdens completely disappear, they can create a counterweight of positive elements, which in turn reduces the influence of stress in their lives.

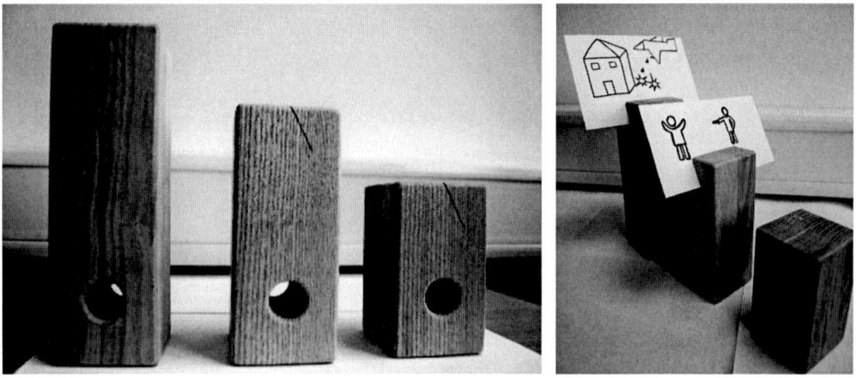

Trauma-Cubes

Trauma-Cubes as a language reduced trauma-therapeutic method have been developed in order to illustrate reactions on traumatic experiences in a tangible way, and in this way to create a direct link to personal resources (Özkan & Belz, 2013). These particular resources shall be elaborated by working with special wooden blocks.

Required material for the methodological procedure:

1. Wooden blocks in three different heights, each with a slit on top and a hole at the bottom (see the figure above);
2. Various index cards;
3. A pen.

In the first step, burdening situations such as the original traumatic situation, triggers or flashbacks are identified on index cards. Once identified, the patient outlines or symbolizes them and organizes them according to a hierarchy. Every situation, which the patient has experienced as traumatic, is being captured on one of the cards. The situation which has been identified as the most incriminating is put into the slit of the biggest block. From there, the less burdening situations are placed into the according medium or small sized blocks. Subsequently the wood blocks are placed in front of the patient. Situations being relevant in the present are placed close to the patient, situations with less current impact are placed more far away.

In the second phase, the patient elaborates with the therapist's help individual resources based on the most burdening situation in the highest wood

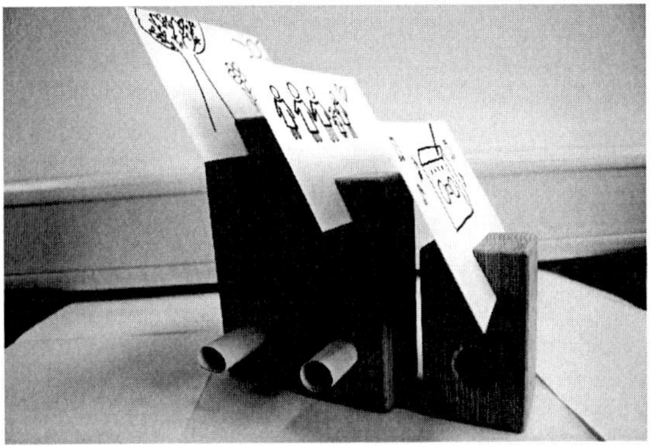

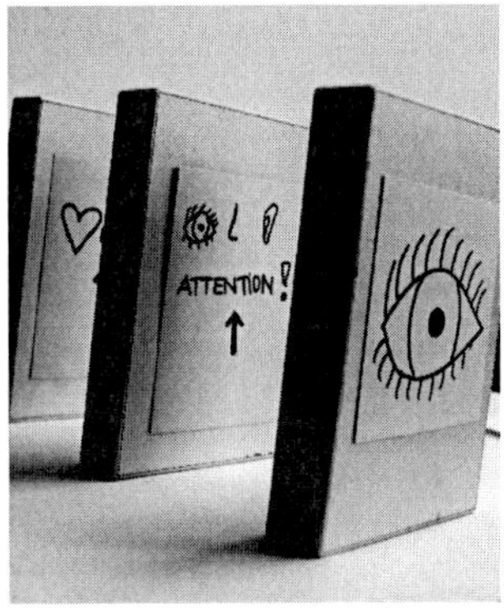

block and outlines them as well. The resources should give the opportunity to cope with this experience and can be anything that is being perceived as helpful, making feel good, activating, etc.

The next step in the process is replacing the index cards with the individual resources cards in the slit on top of the block. With this, the card with the burdening experience is rolled up (with the drawing on the inside) and placed into the hole at the bottom of the block instead.

The same procedure is done in descending order for the other blocks. In this way, an index card with related resources is added to each stressing situation and can replace the burdening card, so that these can be "put away" as a possibility of distancing (p. 208, Özkan & Belz, 2013).

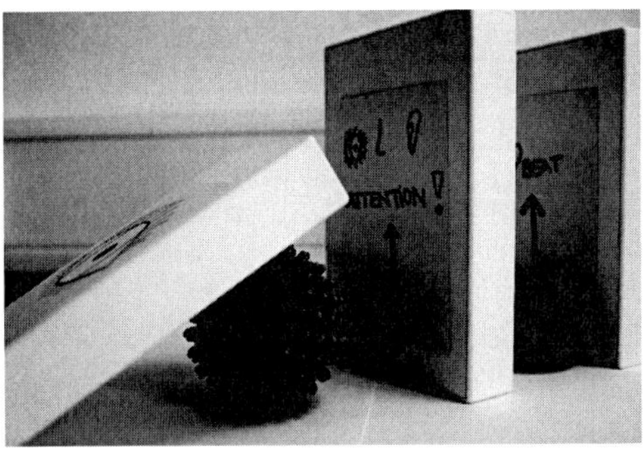

After completing the process, all wooden blocks show personal resources on index cards, which provide strength and help coping with burdening situations. The traumatic experiences are rolled up in the hole at the bottom.

The Chain reaction

The main aim of the chain-reaction method is psychoeducation by illustrating the process of intrusions, flashbacks and subsequent reactions as normal, ordinary biological reactions (Özkan & Belz, 2013). Secondly, resources and possibilities for superior stress tolerance are being detected by using this method.

Required materials for the methodological procedure are:

1. Various wood panels (app. 15x15x2 cm), coated that writing on them with whiteboard-markers is possible (alternatively wood panels with self-adhesive notepads for the labelling);
2. Various personal items from the patient, which either symbolically represent certain skills or are used concretely for skills;
3. a pen.

First, patient and therapist label the wood panels step-by-step what physically happens when he or she experiences flashbacks or intrusions, basing the information from the patient's individual experience. In the beginning, for example, something is being perceived visually or olfactorily (as a trigger) – an eye as a symbol for visual perception can be drawn on the first wood panel. The patient and therapist elaborate symbols for each (bodily) reaction to this trigger (the increase in pulse rate, respiration changes, dilation in the eyes, increased sweating, etc.) and outline each one on a panel. Each labelled wood panel is set exactly in the order of the patients' physical reaction.

It is important to take into account that this process is different for every patient. Because of this, the possibilities for drawing or labelling on the panels are varied. Options include: pictures, thoughts, memories, black outs, when the patient feels himself / herself captured in the past.

It is important to highlight that these are natural processes that are inbuilt, automated physical reactions. Because of this, these reactions may be too fast to perceive or ascertain.

The individual's chain reaction is now illustrated by setting all panels in one line, like dominoes (see the fig. above). To figure out the overwhelming effects of being triggered, the patient or the therapist pushes the first panel, which causes all the wood panels successively to fall. This becomes a symbol for the hardly stoppable chain reaction, which is being triggered in the patient.

After this demonstration of the domino effect, all of the wood panels are set again.

In the next step, patient and therapist try to find out skills, a resource for each step as a change in the process (represented on the wood panels), by which this can be managed or stopped at this very step, e.g. "What can be done to reduce the pulse rate again?" to prevent the next step to fall.

Any item representing possibilities to make reactions controllable may be used to outline a skill on (stones, books, games – everything that stands symbolically for the skill).

Subsequently, the items that are tools to manage the reaction are located between the wood panels and the panel is set a little bit in distance to the next following.

By pushing the first wood panel now, the patient perceives that the following panels do not all automatically fall over, as the items located between the panels hinder the chain reaction. This illustrates that the skills and personal resources (symbolized by the items) can interrupt the chain reaction, and thus, stop the domino effect. In best-case scenario, they are able to prevent the consequences of the chain reaction, such as flashbacks.

References

Agronin, M. (2009). Group therapy in older adults. Current Psychiatry Reports, 11(1), 27–32.

Antonovsky, A. (1996). The salutogenic model as a theory to guide health promotion. Health Promotion International, 11 (1), 11–18.

Belz, M., & Özkan, I. (2013). Ressourcenaktivierende Gruppe für Patienten mit Migrationshintergrund, In: GVS (Ed.), Interkulturelle Suchthilfe – Menschen mit Migrationshintergrund besser verstehen' Partnerschaftlich 03/2013 (S. 10–11). Berlin: GVS-Selbstverlag.

Bermejo, I., Berger, M., Kriston, L., & Härter, M. (2009). Ist Patientenzufriedenheit in der stationären Depressionsbehandlung von der Qualität sprachlicher Deutschkenntnisse abhängig? Psychiatrische Praxis, 36, 279–285.

Bundespsychotherapeutenkammer. (2010). Reformbedarf in der psycho therapeutischen Versorgung von Migranten. Retrieved from http://www.bptk.de/uploads/media/20100614_bptk_standpunkt_pt_versorung_migranten.pdf

Brucks, U. (2004). Der blinde Fleck der medizinischen Versorgung in Deutschland. Migration und psychische Erkrankung. Psychoneuro, 30 (4), 228–231.

Federal Office for Migration and Refugees. (2015). Migrationsbericht 2013. Retrieved from http://www.bamf.de/SharedDocs/Anlagen/DE/Publikationen/Migrationsberichte/migrationsbericht-2013.html

Federal Office for Migration and Refugees. (2008). Sprachliche Integration von Migranten in Deutschland. Retrieved from http://www.bamf.de/SharedDocs/Anlagen/DE/Publikationen/WorkingPapers/wp14-sprachliche-integration.html

Hüther, G. (2004). Die Bedeutung sozialer Erfahrungen für die Strukturierung des menschlichen Gehirns. Welche sozialen Beziehungen brauchen Schüler und Lehrer? Zeitschrift für Pädagogik, 50 (4), 487–495.

Lazarus, R. S. & Folkman, S. (1984). Stress, Appraisal and Coping. New York: Springer.

Leszcz, M. (2004). Group therapy. In: Sadavoy, J., Jarvik, L. F., Grossberg, G. T., Meyers B. S. (Eds.) Comprehensive Textbook of Geriatric Psychiatry: 1023–1054. New York: W.W. Norton and Co.

Liedl, A., Schäfer, U., & Knaevelsrud, C. (2013). Psychoedukation bei posttraumatischen Störungen. Stuttgart: Schattauer Verlag.

Özkan, I. (2013). Ressourcenorientierte traumazentrierte Behandlung von Migranten. In: Körner, W., Irdem, G., Bauer, U. (Eds.). Psycho-soziale Beratung von Migranten. (292–304). Stuttgart: Kohlhammer.

Özkan, I, Belz, M (2013). Ressourcenorientierte traumazentrierte Behandlung von Migranten. In: Feldmann, R. E. Jr. & Seidler, G. H. (Eds.), Traum(a) Migration. (193–220). Gießen: Psychosozial-Verlag.

Özkan, I. & Belz, M. (2014). Neue Wege in der Behandlung von traumatisierten Migranten. Stabilisierung jenseits von Sprache und Traumatherapie. Nervenheilkunde, 6 (405–492), 451–454.

Özkan, I., Belz, M., Oktay, N. (2012). Zusammenhänge von Migration und Stress in Bezug auf das Lernvermögen. In Heise, T., Özkan, I., Golsabahi, S. (Eds.). Integration, Identität, Gesundheit. Beiträge zum 5. Kongress des DTPPP in Klagenfurt 2011 (121–130). Berlin: VWB.

Schouler-Ocak, M., Bretz, H. J., Hauth, I., Heredia Montesinos A., Koch, E., Driessen, M. & Heinz, A. (2010). Patienten mit Migrationshintergrund in

Psychiatrischen Institutsambulanzen – ein Vergleich zwischen Patienten mit türkischer und osteuropäischer Herkunft sowie Patienten ohne Migrationshintergrund. Psychiatrische Praxis, 37, 384–390.
Sachsse, U., Schröder, S., Vogel, V. (2004). Klinisch erfolgreich – Empirisch erfolgreich? Zwischenergebnisse zur Behandlung traumatisierter Patientinnen vom Phänotyp der Borderline-Persönlichkeitsstörung mit selbstverletzendem Verhalten. In: Sachsse, U., Özkan, I., Streeck-Fischer, A. (Eds.) Traumatherapie – Was ist erfolgreich? (42–56). Göttingen: Vandenhoeck & Ruprecht.
Shapiro, F., & Maxfield, L. (2002). Eye movement desensitization and reprocessing (EMDR): Information processing in the treatment of trauma. Journal of Clinical Psychology, 58 (8), 933–946.
Teegen, F. (2000). Psychotherapie der Posttraumatischen Belastungsstörung. Psychotherapeut, 45 (6), 341–349.
Wolf, V., & Özkan, I. (2012). Dolmetschen in der Psychotherapie-Ergebnisse einer Umfrage. Psychotherapeuten- Journal, 4, 325–327

Short CV

Ibrahim Özkan
Information about Ibrahim Özkan are written down at the end of his first article (p. 25)

Maria Belz
Email: m.belz@asklepios.com. Graduated psychologist and in training to become a certified behavioral psychotherapist, she works in the out-patient department of the psychiatric hospital "Asklepios Fachklinikum Göttingen", Rosdorfer Weg 70, 37081 Göttingen, Germany. She is employed in the focus-group for culture, migration, and mental illness. As a certified Trainer she is holding Diversity Seminars.

Access to mental health care for traumatized refugees: Danish perspectives

Marianne Kastrup MD, PhD Copenhagen

Introduction

The Danish population has an increasing proportion of migrants – presently about 450.000 out of 5.25 million. It is however from Europe, that Denmark receives the largest number of migrants as about 53% have a European origin. Approximately 31 % come from Asia including the Middle East. Among those arriving to the country in 2013, 47% came with a EU citizen permit, 26 % came as students, 6 % as part of family unification and only 4% came as asylum seekers (Danish Immigration Office 2013). The origin and number of asylum seekers is reflecting the overall political situation and at present, the countries dominating are Syria and Afghanistan. A study from 2007 carried out by Amnesty International among Danish asylum seekers (Mesmas et al 2008) demonstrated that 45 % had experienced torture and 63 % of these fulfilled the diagnostic criteria for PTSD. Physical symptoms were twice as common and psychological symptoms 2–3 times more common among those who had been tortured compared to the rest.

The geographical distribution of migrants in the country is skewed with particular concentration in certain parts of the larger cities where more than 25 % of the population have a non-Western background.

Historical development of services

In 1973, Amnesty International appealed to the medical profession globally, for help to combat torture and among other things this resulted in the creation of the first medical group in Amnesty International in Denmark, aiming to provide documentation that human rights violation had taken place (Kastrup et al 1987).

Subsequently the group demonstrated that the victims of human rights violation had a number of both physical and psychological symptoms requiring medical interventions. The public health system in Denmark at that time had no focus on this and consequently an initiative was taken to establish treatment facilities, namely the International Rehabilitation and Research Centre for Torture Victims (RCT) in 1983 (Jaranson & Quiroga 2011).

Over the years, Denmark has seen the establishment of a number of other organisations focusing on the treatment of traumatised refugees, as part of the public system and on a more private basis.

Organization of health services

Primary care:

For asylum seekers, the first contact with the Danish healthcare system usually takes place in the asylum centres and is carried out by healthcare personnel employed in these facilities. If found required, a referral may take place to specialized care that is part of the public Danish health services.

For those arriving to the country as illegal migrants they are not entitled to care, but may seek help at a clinic run on a voluntary basis and providing emergency care free of charge.

Once asylum is granted, the contact to health services goes via the GP/family doctors that all citizens with a residence permit are assigned free of charge. The GPs have a key role as coordinator and gateway of all referrals and they may refer the traumatised refugees to psychiatric specialists or to specialised institutions for treatment of traumata.

Secondary care:

The five Regions provide the vast majority of mental health services in the country free of charge and are responsible for the provision of comprehensive psychiatric care.

Specialised treatment to traumatized refugees

Up to about a decade ago, the Danish psychiatric services did not prioritize the treatment of refugees with PTSD. Treatment possibilities for this population were unevenly distributed and long waiting lists the rule. (Even now, the present treatment capacity in the specialised treatment facilities is insufficient).

However, with increasing recognition of the public obligation to provide treatment for this population the Danish National Board of Health did emphasize in its strategic plan for psychiatry that all the five regions should establish specialized services for traumatized refugees as part of the public mental health services and that 1–2 of the Regional services should provide highly specialized services. This is now the case.

Services for traumatised refugees:

Today all Regions provide services including (Kastrup & Dymi 2015):

Capital Region:

The Region provides different treatment facilities. One facility that is part of the public psychiatric services comprises contact with psychiatrist, psychologist and social worker and provides psychopharmacological medication, psychoeducation, structured cognitive therapy and psychosocial support. The treatment is highly manualized, it is individually based and lasts approximately 6 months

Two other organisations in the Capital Region treat traumatised refugees with a contract allowing public funding. Here treatment includes contact with psychologist, social worker, physiotherapist/body therapist, medical doctor (in one of them) and possibility for referral to psychiatrist.

Treatment includes psychotherapy, physiotherapy and psychopharmacological treatment; it may be individual, group or family-oriented and lasts between 6 months and a year.

Zealand Region:

The public institution offers treatment that consists of psychoeducation, individual psychotherapy, body therapy, music therapy, acupuncture and psychosocial support. There is a possibility for referral to a medical doctor for psychopharmacological treatment. Treatment lasts 6–18 months.

Southern Denmark Region:

Treatment is here depending on the bio-psychosocial resources of the patient. Patients with high bio-psychosocial resources are offered initial mentalising psychotherapy, and individual treatment; those with medium bio-psychosocial resources will be offered mentalising psychotherapy and symptom-based group therapy; and those with low bio-psychosocial resources will be offered individual psychoeducation and resource-supportive treatment at home. Treatment combines psychological, somatic and social aspects.

There is a possibility of referral to psychiatrist and psychopharmacological treatment

Middle Denmark Region:

The public institution offers treatment including contact with psychologist, physiotherapist, social worker and contact with a psychiatrist for psychopharmacological treatment. It includes psychotherapy, physiotherapy, psychoeducation, a health issues interview but may also include workshop activities and other social activities. The treatment lasts 4–6 months.

Northern Denmark Region:

Treatment includes contact with a psychologist and physiotherapist, and contact with a social worker and psychiatrist if needed and may include a municipal social rehabilitation offer. The treatment lasts around 9 months.

Discussion

The services provided do have certain similarities but also differences and one may well wonder why it is so in a country of such size that there is no agreement as to what is the best care to offer, and why there are no national guidelines available.

All services have a focus on psychotherapy, on multidisciplinary treatment, on psychosocial counselling and on psychoeducation. However, there are differences as to e.g. the focus on somatic aspects, on physiotherapy, on access to psychiatrist and the availability on group therapy and family therapy.

Several reasons may be given to these differences.

One is political. Each Region has a high degree of autonomy when deciding what healthcare to offer and may have different priorities.

A second reason is a reflection of differences in availability of – in particular psychiatrists – in some areas of the country where a shortage may necessitate other solutions.

A third reason refers to differences in size of the traumatised population of the particular Region.

A fourth reason relates to that different centres nevertheless may have a particular interest or expertise in a certain treatment and historically some treatment initiatives may have started with a non-medical focus.

Finally, we should be aware of that the evidence for effective treatment of traumatised refugees is limited. A Cochrane review concludes that individual trauma-focused cognitive-behavioural therapy, eye movement desensitisation and reprocessing (EMDR), stress management and group Trauma-Focused-Cognitive-Behavioural-Therapy are all effective in the treatment of PTSD. It highlights that trauma-focused treatments are more effective than non-trauma focused treatments (Buhmann 2014).

Perspectives

The current situation vis-à-vis refugees clearly demonstrate that there is an urgent need to optimize services for the traumatized population.

We need robust research focusing on which interventions show the greatest evidence, and is it possible at an early stage to identify factors of significant predictive value for later outcome of a given intervention?

Traumatized refugees are not a homogenous population but differ with respect to a number of factors including educational background, ego-strength, use of coping strategies, language ability, availability of social network, and religious beliefs. Interventions should take this into account.

When this treatment took its start, it was found very relevant to provide services in specialized centres, and not as part of the overall health system. Over the years, we have seen that the therapeutic activities move towards mainstream public mental health services. This development has been beneficial in that it allows mental health services in general to have a larger focus on the impact of trauma as well as cultural matters for the benefit of not just traumatized patients but for all.

References

Danish Immigration Office www.nyidanmark.dk 2013

Masmas TN et al. Asylum seekers in Denmark–a study of health status and grade of traumatization of newly arrived asylum seekers. Medical Group, Amnesty International, Copenhagen, Denmark. Torture 2008; 18: 77–86.

Kastrup M, Lunde I, Ortman J, Genefke I Victimization Inside and Outside the Family: Families of Torture – Consequences and Possibilities for Rehabilitation. PsychCritique. Internat. J. Crit. Psychol. Psychoanal. 1987; 2: 337–349.

Jaranson J, Quiroga, J., Evaluating the services of torture rehabilitation programmes: History and recommendations Torture 2011; 21 nr. 2.

Kastrup M, Dymi K. A therapy model for traumatized refugees in Denmark. In: Schouler-Ocak M. Trauma and Migration. Berlin: Springer Verlag, 2015.

Buhmann C. Traumatized refugees: Morbidity, treatment and predictors of outcome, PhD thesis defended/approved by the Univ. of Copenhagen on 9.4.2014.

Short CV

Marianne C. Kastrup

2014–2015 Consultant to Dignity – Danish Institute against Torture, Copenhagen

2001–2014 Head and consultant to Competence Centre Transcultural Psychiatry, Psychiatric Center Ballerup, Copenhagen University Hospital, Denmark.
MK is the author/co-author of more than 100 peer-review articles, 15 books, and more than 80 book-chapters.
She has presented more than 300 international abstracts.
MK has wide range of experience in international organizations. She has been a member of the World Psychiatric Association Executive Committee, been the Zonal Representative Northern Europe, WPA and chair of the Transcultural Section. She is currently a Member of the Board of European Psychiatric Association and was for years Secretary General, European Psychiatric Association. She is currently the Treasurer of the World Association for Social Psychiatry.
She has for many years served as a Member Expert Advisory Panel on Mental Health, WHO

Mental Health Promotion – How could it help in dealing with Posttraumatic Stress Disorder

Hartmut Berger

Health promotion and especially mental health promotion is still a frequently neglected area in psychiatry. In the treatment of acute diseases one will not find recommendations for mental health promotion at all because our thinking is still stamped by diagnosing and treating of symptoms and not more. Therefore, the human being behind the disease is often falling into oblivion. However, there is much evidence that health promoting strategies are very useful in coping especially with severe mental disorders such as posttraumatic stress disorders (Berger 2015). This disease has a high and may be growing prevalence in Europe especially as a consequence of war and migration. Currently the estimated life time prevalence of PTSD adds up to 1 – 7 % in Europe (Darvez-Bornoz 2008). 30 % of untreated patients show symptoms after 10 years (Kessler et al 1995) and 10–20 % come down with a chronic course (Hidalgo, Davidson 2000). Furthermore, PTSD is very often associated with other mental disorders. Conventional guidelines recommend for example to care for a safe environment, to do supportive psychotherapy, cognitive behaviour therapy, exposition therapy, Eye Movement Desensitization and Reprocessing, psychoeducation and psychopharmacotherapy (Flatten et al 2011). But these strategies – as worthful as they are – don't meet the patients needs for mental health promotion.

Mental health promotion is based on the concept of salutogenesis. Salutogenesis is researching the factors and interdependecies, which are responsible to keep persons healthy inspite of trauma. Thus far mental health is not a state but a process. Salutogenesis is investigating factors and ressources, which promote this process. The core of salutogenesis is the sense of coherence (SOC). The SOC encompasses 3 dimensions, which are essential for successful coping with traumatic life events: comprehensibility, manageability and meaningfulness (Antonovsky 1987). In this respect Mental Health promotion is a process, which should give people more self determination about their health and thus strenghten their health. With other words: "To get global physical, mental and social wellbeing it's necessary, that individuals meet their needs, realize their hopes and desires and are able to master their environment" (Bengel 2003). Mental health promotion is using different strategies such as improving empowerment, implementing shared decision making, implementing codetermination, promotion of self efficacy, promotion of sense of coherence, promotion of resilience and promotion of recovery. In the following these strategies should briefly be defined.

Empowerment is a "process to gain self control and influence on environment" (Segal 1995). The aim of empowerment is that "individuals have a low threshold access to information about the illness and it's treatment options. They have options, are able to realize their needs and willing to take responsibility for themselves" (Naidoo 2003).

Shared decision making means a comprehensive education and the inclusion of patients options into the process of decision making. Thus the therapy is based on an informed consent of patients. A step further is to deal with codetermination, which means that the patient's opinion has the same sigificance as the therapist's intention.

Self efficacy is the strongest psychological amplifier of human action (Bandura 1977). Thus strengthening self efficacy is a powerful instrument in mental health promotion.

The same applies to resilience, which means the "ability to overcome stressful life events stronger and with more ressources than before" (Walsh 1988). Even if we don't know the causes of resilience in the life time, we have possibilities to reinforce the resilience especially with an appropriate handling of PTSD.

To promote the sense of coherence means to work out stategies of understanding the trauma and managing the consequences as well as helping to find a new sense of life inspite of the trauma.

The process of recovery is an active process which encompasses the elements: 1. the return to normality, 2. the restoration of health and 3. learning useful messages from the trauma (Schmolke u Amering 2007). Recovery includes hope, self control, active participation, change potential, optimism, creativity, holistic point of view (Bradstreet 2011) and includes at one hand personal recovery which means hope, identity, personal responsibility, meaningfulness and on the other hand clinical recovery which encompasses symptom reduction, improvement of social functioning, successful risk management and relapse prevention (Slade 2009).

To bring the described strategies into practice, it's necessary to change the attitude of therapeutic settings. One possibility is to define standards of mental health promotion as the task force health promoting psychiatric services did. The task force is a working group implemented by the Health Promoting Hospitals network (HPH), which is sponsored by the World Health Organization containing more than 600 hospitals all over the world. The task force composed standards which are closely related to the general standards of the Health Promoting Hospitals Network in consideration of the special demands of mental health services. In accordance with the Vienna Recommendations deriving from the Budapest declaration (WHO 1986), health promoting hospitals oblige themselves to recognize and honor the following basic principles: 1.The individual person should be the focus of their endeavors; 2. They should orient themselves to a holistic concept of health and disease; 3.They should orient their activities to human dignity, equality and solidarity, always in respect of the varying needs of the different cultural groups within the community; 4. They should orient themselves to the well-being of the patients, families and staff and obligate themselves to the protection of the environment; 5. They should use their resources wisely in accordance with the measure of their contribution to health and should apply their efforts to the active cooperation and networking with other health services (Pelikan et al 1998).

The solution to these tasks demands novel instruments that surmount the traditional way of thought. The concept of mental health promotion is particularly suitable in that: It focuses upon the individual person in the totality of their life references; it promotes the active participation and self-responsibility of the patients, their families and the staff; it aims to support the available and natural resources; it requires a holistic view that accords the prevention of and active coping with disease, as well as the improvement of the quality of life the same value as the treatment; it supports healthy working conditions for the staff, i.e. the organization ensures the establishment and implemenation of a comprehensive human resource strategy that includes the development and training of staff in mental health promotion skills and it ensures the involvement of staff in decisions impacting on the staff's working environment; it aims to improve the communication among the staff in order to enhance the quality of life in the workplace by implementing measures of further education and training in areas relevant to mental health promotion; it focuses upon the entirety of the health services field in the sense of setting approaches, as well as upon their inclusion in the social framework, and enhances the communication and cooperation of all institutions active in the field; it understands it health services as learning organizations, through which education, training and self-reflection can change existing routines, tailoring them as needed and continually to keep pace with the changing needs of their users; it is an instrument suitable for integration and promotion of the dialogue among the various schools of psychiatric thought (Berger, Paul 1998).

In the framework of these standards procedures for mental health promotion on an individual level should be: 1. The assessment of needs for mental health promotion, this assessment should be done at the first contact and be aware of sensitivity to social, cultural and religious background. 2. The patients should be informed about diagnosis, prognosis and treatment possibilities 3. A patient advisor should be offered. 4. Evidence based interventions for mental health promotion like mindful based procedures, stress management, support of self-help, improvement of the sense of coherence, including family members and partners in therapeutic alliances like multifamilyintervention (Berger 2014) should be obligatory parts of the treatment. These are only some examples of mental health promoting strategies. There are much more activities thinkable. Crucial is not what is done but how it's done.

Rethinking therapeutic settings in the described way and embedding conventional therapeutic standards in the framework of mental health promotion will improve the therapeutic results, patient satisfaction, their ability to cope even with threatening life events and will improve resilience, self efficacy, the recovery process and last but not least the quality of life of patients who experienced post traumautic stress disorders

References

Berger H 2015. Die Förderung seelischer Gesundheit. In: Rössler W, Ajdacic-Gross V (Hrsg) Prävention psychischer Störungen. Kohlhammer Stuttgart

Darves-Bornoz JM, Alonso J, de Girolamo G, de Graaf R, Haro JM, Kovess-Masfety V, ?Lépine JP, Nachbaur G, Negre-Pages L, Vilagut G, Gasquet Is 2008. Main traumatic events in Europe: PTSD in the ESEMeD Survey. Journal of Traumatic Stress 21:5, 455–462

Flatten G, Gast U, Hofmann A, Knaevelsrud Ch, Lampe A, Liebermann P, Maercker A, Reddemann L, Wöller W 2011. S3 – Leitlinie Posttraumatische Belastungsstörung. Trauma & Gewalt 3: 202–210

Kessler R C, Sonnega A, Bromet E, Hughes M & Nelson C B 1995. Posttraumatic stress disorder in the National Comorbidity Survey. Archives of General Psychiatry 52 (12), 1048–1060

Hidalgo RB Davidson JR 2000. Posttraumatic stress disorder: epidemiology and health- related considerations. J Clin Psychiatry: 61 Suppl 7:5–13

Antonovsky A 1987. Unraveling the Mystery of Health. Jossey Bass San Francisco

Bengel J, Herwig J 2003. Gesundheitsförderung in der Rehabilitation. In: Jerusalem M, Weber H (Hrsg.) Psychologische Gesundheitsförderung. Göttingen Bern Toronto Seattle: Hogrefe

Segal SP, Silverman C, Temkin T. 1995. Measuring empowerment in client run self-help agencies. Community Mental Health Journal; 31:215–227

Naidoo J, Wills J 2000. Lehrbuch der Gesundheitsförderung. Gamburg: Verlag für Gesundheitsförderung.

Bandura A 1977. Self-efficacy: Toward a Unifying Theory of Behavioral Change. Psychological Review 84: 191–215

Walsh F 1998. Strengthening Family Resilience. New York. Guilford Press

Amering M, Schmolke M 2012. Recovery Das Ende der Unheilbarkeit. Bonn: Psychiatrie-Verlag

Bradstreet S 2011. Scottish recovery network. www.scottishrecovery.net. Zugriff am 11.08.2015

Slade M 2009. Personal Recovery and Mental Illness: A guide for Mental Health Professionals. Cambridge: University Press

WHO 1986. Ottawa Charter for Health Promotion. Geneva: WHO

Pelikan, J.M., Garcia-Barbero, M., Lobnig, H., Krajic, K. 1998. Pathways to a Health Promoting Hospital, Gamburg, G. Conrad

Berger, H., Paul, R 1998. The Health Promoting Hospital – What is the Difference? Experiences from the Philippshospital Pilot Hospital Project in Riedstadt, in: Pelikan, J.M., Garcia-Barbero, M., Lobnig, H., Krajic, K. (ed.): Pathways to a Health Promoting Hospital, Gamburg, G. Conrad, pp. 71–94.

Short CV

Hartmut Berger

1974–1975 Physician at the first drug councelling center Frankfurt;

1976–1977 Resident University Hospital Frankfurt;

1978–1980 Resident Neurological Departement St. Katharinen Krankenhaus Frankfurt;

1981–1990 head of department Psychiatric Clinic Offenbach;

1991–2014 Medical Director Psychiatric Clinic Riedstadt;

since 2004 Professor of Psychioatry Technical University Darmstadt;

since 2010 lectureship Goethe University Frankfurt;

1998–2014 coordinator task force on health Promoting Psychiatric Services on behalf of Health Promoting Hospitals Network sponsored by WHO Europe

Is psychotherapy needed for unsuccessful asylum applicants forced to return to their country?

Abdelhak Elghezouani

Mental health issues with asylum seekers and the increasingly severe treatment of the unsuccessful asylum applicants involve significant effects on the health services and the professionals in terms of ethics, resources and attitudes and consequently on the applicants themselves.

From the point of view of the professional in mental health, the problems presented by the unsuccessful applicants and those waiting for repatriation and granted minimal assistance are marked by a deep psychological distress often causing psychic, somatic or psychosomatic breakdown.

This psychic suffering is not always related to a pre-existent psychiatric pathology or to consequences of violence or ill treatment but strongly seems to be the direct and catastrophic consequence of some determinants, collective and individual, political, social and historical. In fact, the mental health professional can only note that, first of all, the "crisis" is not "in" the individual, but in the environment in which this individual evolves/moves.

However, the therapeutic attitude towards an individual reduced to an infra human statute requires to identify the subjective and objectives factors responsible for this distress and to act against the noxious character of these pathogenic factors for both protagonists of the therapeutic encounter. Helping or healing appears then to be a limit-situation with the danger of being overwhelmed by feelings of persecution, powerlessness, guilt, etc., for both protagonists. Avoiding these feelings can also lead to attitudes, movements and behaviours which are not, sometimes, less violent, dreadful and destructive, than the situation itself, proving detrimental to the therapist and/or to the patient.

For the unsuccessful asylum seekers who did not forsake psychological help, the distress is accompanied by a loss of psychic boundaries leading to laying bare old and/or current defaults through the loss of a minimal social status; undoubtedly provoked by of the disappearance of a life plan. This objective failure is doubled by a self-coherence bankruptcy: Odyssey replacing the migratory plan. The collapse is worsened by the incapacity of the mental health services to continue to be effective.

Psychosocial distress following the bankruptcy of self-coherence leads to, at best, a logic of day to day survival for the more enduring and most adventurous individuals; and in the worst case, a depersonalization and a derealisation, feelings of persecution, loss of self-confidence and trust others and in the world.

"Pathologies", or more exactly ways of adjustment, are then pathologies acting out, psychosomatic pathologies or pathologies of anaclitic collapses or of the parcelling out of oneself. The mental health professional may be overwhelmed by defence and reactive movements such as refusal, cynicism, identification to the aggressor, powerlessness, etc. By their psychosocial effects, the consequences of the refusal of asylum application and the threat of deportation, dare the professionals to imagine new postures, ethical and relational, theoretical and therapeutic.

Today, many individuals excluded from a "social contract" and entered to a kind of a desperate and destroying wandering, are sometimes referred by other professionals or come of their own volition knocking on our door and challenging mental health professionals with the vehemence of their tragic despair. Part of these individuals are patients, claiming either more or something entirely different to psychiatric and/or psychotherapeutic assistance; or are willing to talk to someone else than their therapist; or with their therapist but on more time that s/he can grant to them. An eventual current therapy showing its inadequacy confronted with a supplication not only overflowing, but also devouring and unrealistic, and apparently exceeding our therapeutic capacity. Consequently, it becomes necessary to think of new goals the psychotherapies granted to both asylum seekers and unsuccessful asylum seekers threatened with deportation to their country of origin.

Exile is then to be conceived as the materialization of a life plan based on what A. Adler calls "a fictional final goal": for example, that of the satisfaction of the basic needs, or the political, spiritual, narcissistic ones, etc. The other side of the problem is the failure to achieve this life plan in the home country, among family and relatives now left behind and abandoned. The migration plan and its' failure should be conceived as what they are: intimate, private and collective issues and plans, implemented throughout the journey: a geographical change, a confrontation with the other, frustrating or generous, a confrontation with what is different or unknown, with luck and risk, etc. But one should not forget to address the strong feelings of hopelessness and powerlessness of the therapist. Exiled from himself or herself on a new and strange land, missing his or her reference marks and his or her usual tools. The "social counter-transference" may also explain this stroke: unconsciously feeling responsible of an injustice.

If we forsake this assumption: that of the failure and the loss of self-coherence through the loss and the failure of the migratory plan of the patient, it will not be possible any more to reach and mobilize the interiority of the subject, his/her internal world and its' dynamics, its' actors and its' objects emerging in broad day-light exactly when the object evades. Similarly, for the therapist, the failure or the absence of a symptoms-oriented therapeutic project, and the underhand effects of the social counter-transference can constitute a basis making a new "therapeutic" plan possible.

Boundaries should thus be rehabilitated, especially when they allow access to interiority and in giving shape to "unshaped" thoughts, emotions and actions and to support the capacity of symbolization when it was eroded and had even disappeared.

However, when the object evades, for example the migratory project, the "object-relation", in Freudian words, is naked and the lifestyle according to Adler becomes as much source of symptoms as source of resources for change. Who among therapists has not felt the strong rush to call a lawyer or start drafting an umpteenth report, vain and useless, exhausting and tiresome as if forced to hide an obscene and provocative subjectivity which is breaking the perfect image of the innocent victim of an unjust fate. A victim with whom support or accompaniment was so quiet, gratifying, reducing the apparent symptoms, by the magic power of solidarity and consolation but never reaching the major stake.

It is thus necessary to keep an inward view before a disorganizing catastrophe (e.g. a non prepared forced repatriation) happens, for the patient and for the therapist. Or for better calling upon this subjectivity the day the catastrophe comes and when confrontation to reality cannot be avoided any more.

What is this object which evaded when the migratory plan is destroyed? Do we know anything about it? Even after many sessions of symptoms focused therapy? Generally, we know nothing or very little, because the sessions were saturated with issues brought about by an objective reality, striking, but also providing feelings of safety, achievement and high morality.

These are few hypotheses to counteract negative feelings when confronted with situations where we cannot neither give satisfaction to demands from our patients nor change anything in their concrete situation.

To propose an operational theory, is to also necessary to consider the collective, social, political issues, and to analyze their determinism on the individual's psychic life. In a certain way, a direct correspondence should be established between, on the one hand, the collective dynamics and historicity and, on the other hand, their private "image" such as they appear in clinical work (emotional stakes; debts, merits and loyalties; objective and subjective needs).

The failure of the migratory plan is also a collectively catastrophic event because the project was the project of a group and was conceived as a solution for a group and for narrowly interdependent people. It is also the failure of an attempt at self-emancipation based on an individual. Taking this into consideration appears to be the only way to reach the subjectivity of the patient; the loyalties, debts, mandates and merits attaching him to his groups of membership and nurturing his imaginary.

We choose a transdiagnostic approach as we consider that these patients have to deal with pathogenic strong feelings of frustration, fear, shame, etc. stemming from social conditions, used in a broad sense. We also assume the existence and the activation of mechanisms and strategies of adjustment to unsatisfied needs both in the country of origin and in their current situation. These strong negative feelings put into action particular cognitive, behavioural, emotional and interpersonal strategies deeply rooted and constructed in the biography of the patient.

Our first hypothesis conceives their symptoms as the expression of unsatisfied needs and of unfulfilled purposes of the patient, his family or even his community. We therefore have to deal with idiosyncratic, existential, collective, political and cultural constructions making it possible to commit in a psychotherapeutic work. We draw from Adlers' conception that the individual is embedded in the social context where s/he was raised and where s/he grew up.

Our second hypothesis conceives their symptoms as the expression of what Adler called their style of life or lifestyle which is the way an individual reacts and adjusts to his/her environment in an attempt to achieve his/her self-coherence. In other words, unsatisfied needs challenge their self-coherence and put their life style into action.

The third hypothesis is that discovering their life style and how they conceive their self-coherence will enable them to understand and /or change their way of facing life challenges, including the current challenge they have to deal with, and even forming new values and new life purposes.

So the focus of the therapy will be the migration plan and the social (in a broad sense) circumstances where it took shape. Moreover, we assume that this approach should be proposed to all asylum seekers as they are confronted to new life conditions, sometimes to a harshness challenging their life style and their self-coherence. The asylum proceedings are bound to take many years, making them living a long period of uncertainty. More than fifty per cent of applicants will be unsuccessful and will be confronted with the threat of being deported to their country or even be forced to return.

Short CV

Psychologist at Association APPARTENANCES. Consultation Psychothérapeutique pour Migrants. Rue des Terreaux, 10. CH 1003 Lausanne (Switzerland)
E-mail: a.elghezouani@appartenances.ch; aelghezouani@hotmail.com

Mental Health of Traumatized Refugees and Asylum Seekers in Germany

Altunoz U, Machleidt W, Graef-Calliess I.T.

Germany has always been an important host country for asylum seekers. Since 1953 4.1 million people applied for Asylum in Germany and 77.4% of them since 1990 were applied. The highest application rate was in 1992 (438.191). In 2014 202.834 persons applied for Asylum. There was an increase of %59.7 when compared with 2013. Countries of origin of those applicants were Syria, Serbia, Eritrea, Albania, Afghanistan, Kosovo, Bosnia-Herzegovina, Macedonia, Somalia, and Iraq. Federal Office for Migration & Refugees is responsible for the process of asylum application.

Access to health care for asylum seekers in Germany is regulated by the national Law on Services for Asylum Seekers (AsylBLG sections 4 and 6), which covers emergency medical care, treatment for acute and painful conditions, and care during pregnancy and childbirth, vaccinations and some other measures which are deemed to be "essential" to preserve health. Therefore, it is difficult for them to reach proper treatment options for chronic diseases and psychiatric trauma. Social Welfare Office often denied reimbursement for such conditions. The asylum seekers can go directly to the emergency services. However, for any other urgent health problems they should personally take a document from Social Welfare Office and in addition to that, referral of a physician is required. Due to these administrations; asylum seekers and refugees may not see a physician until their health has deteriorated sharply, so that they constitute an emergency. This problem is long known and has been mentioned by civil society organizations and health professionals via initiatives ranging from political campaigns to the provision of solidarity health-care services (Schneider et al 2014).

Information about health status and provision of the health care to asylum seekers is not captured by German routine health information system. There is yet no systematic overview on the health status of and health-care provision to asylum seekers in Germany. Especially there is a paucity of research concerning mental health of the asylum seekers. The international systematic reviews on the prevalence of mental health disorders among asylum seekers, none list any studies conducted in Germany (Schneider et al 2014). That can be due to lack of studies and/or the strikt inclusion criteria of those reviews.

Although, over the last 20 years, an increasing number of investigations into the mental health of individual migrant groups have been published in Germany, there are still only limited data on the health status of asylum seekers and refugees (Machleidt & Sieberer 2013). Many authors have assumed that in comparison to other migrant groups, asylum seekers and refugees have a more impaired general state of health, both physical and mental (e.g. Fazel et al 2005, Gerritsen et al 2006, Maier et al 2010). The results of international research indicate that asylum seekers and those whose asylum applications have been rejected show higher rates of pre-migratory traumatic experience and, accordingly, often have mental disorders associated with trauma (Robjant et al 2009). Along with depressive disorders, somatoform pain disorders (Maier et al 2010) and anxiety disorders, post-traumatic stress disorders contribute most strongly to the increased mental morbidity observed in asylum seekers and refugees (Fazel et al 2005). A meta-analysis showed that the prevalence rate for depression was almost twice as high for refugees and asylum seekers as for so-called "migrant workers" (Lindert et al 2009)

German studies on the subject are very few, most of them written in German and have small samples. Gabel et al (2006) searched PTSD among asylum seekers during the asylum interview process and found that 40 of the 76 asylum seekers had PTSD (40%). Sieberer et al (2011) investigated expert reports of 62 asylum seekers and found that 82.3% of the asylum seekers reported on traumatization. PTSD was the most common diagnosis (74.1%), followed with depressive disorders (ICD-10: F32.x in

33.9 % and ICD-10: F33.x in 25.9 %). Suicidal tendency was found in 56.5 % of the asylum seekers. Von Beutel et al (2007) studied long term effects of being a refugee in a representative community sample and found that former refugees reported reduced quality of life, they suffered more often from panic attacks, were compromised in their health and well-being. Gavranidou et al (2008) investigated psychological symptoms of the refugee children and adolescents (11–17 years) in München. Those refugees report high numbers of emotional and behavioral symptoms and significant correlations were found between exile-related family stressors and current psychological symptoms. Muhtz et al (2011) searched long-term consequences of flight and expulsion during childhood in 502 participants from the former German eastern territories who were displaced as children at the end of World War II (at the age of 5–12 years). 31.5% participants diagnosed with full PTSD, and 33.7% fulfilled the criteria of a current partial PTSD. Participants with PTSD reported a significantly reduced quality of life. That study is very important because it demonstrates the long-term consequences of flight and expulsion during childhood in aging former refugee children more than 60 years later. Nika et al (2000) reported a case of 18 year old Croat refugee with a first episode schizophrenia and discussed the German laws for foreigners as a possible factor for the maintenance of the disease. Short residence permits, the release of the professional discretion to the authorities, deficient information about the laws and the unclear situation in the native country of the patients can lead to a worst course and prognosis of the disease.

There are many civil society organisations, clinics, associations and networks which are dealing with the issue of the health/mental health of the asylum seekers and refugees in Germany. And of course not all the practical work (especially the optimistic ones) could be reflected to the scientific studies. By 1st March 2015 there was a change in the law for asylum seekers and refugees. After 15 months (previously was 4 years) asylum seekers and refugees have the opportunity to have a health insurance card. By this means the bureaucratic procedures will be shorter although the scope of the health care provision stays the same.

And last but not the least! What are we doing? We offer in Klinikum Wahrendorff Transcultural Psychiatry & Psychotherapy Outpatient Clinic special office hours for traumatized refugees in Hannover, Germany. The components of those office hours are culture sensitive asessment, psychiatric emergency care, if necessary referral to our day clinic or other psychiatric services and support by social workers. Besides the individual psychotherapeutic support and psychopharmacological approaches, speech-reduced trauma oriented group therapies are applied in cooperation with Asklepios Clinic-Göttingen.

References

Fazel, M., Wheeler, J., & Danesh, J. 2005. Prevalence of serious mental disorder in 7,000 refugees resettled in western countries: A systematic review. Lancet, 365(9467), 1309–1314.

Gäbel, U., Ruf, M., Schauer, M., Odenwald, M., & Neuner, F. 2006. Prävalenz der Posttraumatischen Belastungsstörung (PTSD) und Möglichkeiten der Ermittlung in der Asylverfahrenspraxis. Zeitschrift für Klinische Psychologie und Psychotherapie, 35, 12–20.

Gavranidou, M., Niemiec, B., Magg, B., Rosner, R.. 2008. Traumatische Erfahrungen, aktuelle Lebensbedingungen im Exil und psychische Belastung junger Flüchtlinge. Kindheit und Entwicklung, 17 (4), 224–231.

Gerritsen, A. A., Bramsen, I., Deville', W., van Willigen, L. H., Hovens, J. E., & van der Ploeg, H. M. 2006. Physical and mental health of Afghan, Iranian and Somali asylum seekers and refugees living in the Netherlands. Social Psychiatry and Psychiatric Epidemiology, 41, 18–26.

Lindert, J., Ehrenstein, O. S., Priebe, S., Mielck, S., & Brahler, E. 2009. Depression and anxiety in labor migrants and refugees: A systematic review and meta-analysis. Social Science and Medicine, 69, 246–257.

Machleidt W, Sieberer M. From Kraepelin to a modern and integrative scientific discipline: the development oftranscultural psychiatry in Germany. Transcult Psychiatry. 2013 Dec; 50(6): 817–40. doi: 10.1177/1363461513508597.

Maier T, Schmidt M, Mueller J. 2010. Mental health and healthcare utilization in adult asylum seekers. Swiss Medical Weekly, 140.

Muhtz C, von Alm C, Godemann K, Wittekind C, Jelinek L, Yassouridis A, Kellner M. [Long-term consequences of flight and expulsion in former refugee children]. Psychother Psychosom Med Psychol. 2011 May; 61(5): 233–8. doi: 10.1055/s-0031-1275341.

Nika E, Briken P, Yagdiran O, Gottwalz E, Krausz M. 2000. [Current German laws for foreigners as a contributory factor in the treatment of a first-time acute schizophrenic episode]. Psychiatr Prax. Oct; 27(7): 357–8.

Robjant K, Hassan R, Katona C. 2009. Mental health implications of detaining asylum seekers: Systematic review. British Journal of Psychiatry, 194, 306–312.

Schneider C, Mohsenpour A, Joos S, Bozorgmehr K. 2014. Health status of and health-care provision to asylum seekers in Germany: protocol for a systematic review and evidencemapping of empirical studies. Syst Rev.; 3: 139. Published online 2014 November 29.

Sieberer M, Ziegenbein M, Eckhardt G, Machleidt W, Calliess I. T. 2011. Psychiatrische Begutachtung im Asylverfahren. Psychiatrische Praxis, 38(1), 38–44.

Von Beutel ME, Decker O, Brähler E. [Quality of life and distress among former refugees – a representative community survey of Germans born before 1946]. Z Psychosom Med Psychother. 2007; 53(3): 203–15.

Short CV

Umut Altunoz, M.D., is a psychiatrist & psychotherapist and researcher in Wahrendorff Clinic, Center of Transcultural Psychiatry & Psychotherapy, Hannover, Germany. He was graduated from Hacettepe University Faculty of Medicine (Ankara, Turkey) and specialized on psychiatry and psychotherapy in Ankara University School of Medicine, Department of Psychiatry. His main areas of interest are transcultural psychiatry, anxiety disorders and geriatric psychiatry. E-Mail: ualtunoz@gmail.com

Wielant Machleidt, Prof. Dr. med., is a Professor emeritus of Social Psychiatry at Hannover Medical School (MHH) and was the head of the Department of Social Psychiatry and Psychotherapy from 1994–2007. He is a specialist in social and cultural psychiatry and, in addition, for psychotherapy and psychoanalysis.

Iris Tatjana Graef-Calliess, Prof. Dr. med, is the head of the Transcultural Psychiatry and Psychotherapy Department of the Wahrendorff Clinic, Hannover, Germany. She is the vice-Chair of Section Cultural Psychiatry of the European Psychiatric Association (EPA) and of the Section Intercultural Psychiatry & Psychotherapy of the German Psychiatric Association (DGPPN).

Transcultural aspects of psychotherapy with couples

Mechthild Gesmann MD Herford

The number of marriages with partners from different countries is continuously increasing but knowledge about how binational relationships work is still sparse.

The vast majority of research into relationship satisfaction of couples from different backgrounds has been conducted in the context of the United States. In 2014 the Netherlands 'Interdisciplinary Demographic Institute' (NIDI) examined whether relationship satisfaction differs between binational and uninational couples. Additionaly they investigated couple characteristics that might affect relationship satisfaction. The results revealed that EU nationals in a binational union reported higher relationship satisfaction compared to individuals in a uninational union. **1**

Dutch nationals in a binational relationship did not report higher satisfaction levels compared to those in uninational unions but the migrants did. The investigation found that place of living, personal history and personality influence one's relationship satisfaction.

Furthermore, investigating the interaction effect of couple status with children, the analysis revealed that individuals in binational unions with children are less happy compared to those in uninational relationships. This seems to be especially true for native individuals in such partnerships. For binational unions, having children might thus be even more challenging compared to the native population. This could be explained by possible conflicts concerning the visions on and attitudes towards child-bearing and -rearing in binational relationships. Native people in binational relationships might compare their child-bearing and -rearing practices with those of surrounding families and friends and perceive differences. It is also possible that they receive more negative feedback from their family and friends on the way they raise their children, if they consider such practices deviant from the general 'Dutch'norm. EU partners might be less exposed to such negative feedback due to the geographical distance to their relatives and friends in the home country. **2**

Relationship satisfaction is influenced by a variety of factors. These refer to social relationships transgressing the boundaries of the romantic relationship as well. The availability of social support from the wider familial and friendship network is positively related to relationship satisfaction.

Social support is associated with reduced distress experience. Attachment theory (J. Bowlby 1969,1988) states that seeking and maintaining a sense of emotional connection with significant others is an innate, primary motivating principle in human beings across their life span. The physical or representational presence of attachment person provides a sense of comfort and security, while the perceived inaccessibility of such person creates distress. In 2009, S.L. Master found that the presence of a partner's picture reduces experimentally induced pain. **3** Simply viewing a loved one's picture can have pain-attenuating effects and simple reminders of loved ones may be sufficient to engender feelings of support.

A safe connection with an attachment person strengthens the ability to take the emotional risk of reaching out empathically to and providing support for others as well as coping with conflict and stress. The more connected we are, the more separate and different we can be. Health in this model is perceived sense of interdependency. **4**

In many distressed relationships, partners are caught in cycles of critical demanding and defensive withdrawal, both in general and in sexual interactions.

Understanding love as attachment provides an image of optimal healthy relatedness and optimal healthy sexuality. In a secure relationship emotional responsiveness, tender touch and erotic playfulness can all come together. Stern (2004) observes that secure lovers are attuned to each other, sensing each other's inner state and intention and responding to each other like an empathic mother does to her baby. In these moments, emotional safety shapes physical synchrony and physical synchrony embodies emotional safety (Johnson 2008, 2009).

In our psychotherapeutic work we use the psychodynamic concept of Positive Psychotherapy (PPT, Nossrat Peseschkian, since 1968). This humanistic psychotherapeutic concept emphasizes the impact of culture and diversity of humans. In the conceptual framework of Positive Psychotherapy, it is described that different cultures deal with a lot of phenomena of life using different strategies of problem solving. **5** Peseschkian gave examples such as choice of partner, handling of money, death or mourning, meaning of work, meaning of the body and many more.

For example, a couple might live in a binational situation (Jamaican – German). The wife will judge situations different from her German husband for example the following: I won't take my time to meet others versus: I will always take my time to meet others. The conflict situation develops on the basis of different cultural concepts on the issues of time and contact. Obviously the conflict of the couple can be described in a psychodynamic way. However, a cross-cultural dimension is needed to explain it efficiently. The individual concepts of time and contact become the source of conflict because of a current context of cultural difference. The wife once says: At the beginning of our relationship both of us had to study a new culture. According to a psychodynamic psychotherapeutic concept the partnership's situation can be described as a conflict situation (autonomy – dependence). In Positive Psychotherapy the conflict situation is described with conflict contents in terms of primary and secondary capabilities, based on the capabilities of loving and knowing.

When it comes to problem solving strategies we can name the following behavioural attributes: punctuality, cleanliness, order, obedience, politeness, honesty, loyalty, justice, industry/achievement, thrift, dependability, exactness, conscientiousness, love, patience, sexuality, trust, confidence, hope, faith, doubt, certainty, and unity. We label these behavioural attributes as actual capabilities because they are rooted in the human being as capabilities and are actually effective in day-to-day life. **6**

The actual capabilities can be divided into primary and secondary capabilities. On the basis of the primary capabilities, the secondary capabilities find their emotional resonance: If you don't clean up your room, it means you don't love me anymore. Just as a steady stream of droplets can eventually hollow out a stone, so the day-to-day-experiences with the actual capabilities create areas of reduced resistance. These are predestined to cause conflicts and psychic and psychosomatic disorders.

The actual capabilities can be realized in an unlimited number of different attitudes, values, experiences, and behavioural patterns. The concepts (for example, “Orderliness is half of life”; “If you have something, you are something”; “What will people say?” et cetera) however, are the situational, group-specified or personality-linked characterizations of these actual capabilities. **7**

On the other hand, the capabilities of dealing with distress and conflicts are helpful and a necessary part of a person with regard to resources.

Mrs. S., a 62-year-old woman asked for consultation. She had been working as a secretary for more than 30 years. Grown up in Jamaica and Great Britain she married her husband in 1978. Her husband, 63 years old, grew up in Germany and worked as a teacher until he retired in 2009 (anxiety disorder, depression). After a mobbing situation at her working place Mrs. N. had developed a pronounced anxiety about being good enough and of being accepted as person. Keeping her distance to the conflict field, she succeeded in finding self-esteem and security. Their partnership was a very strong resource. Mr. S. accompanied his wife each time she came to the practice of her doctor. He used the time for himself, relaxing in the recreation room by listening to slow music lying on a waterbed. Several times we talked in a joint session. Preparing an interview concerning the capabilities of their relationship both partners filled the Wiesbaden Inventory for Positive Psychotherapy and Family Therapy WIPPF, and in the next session we discussed the results.

In family therapy, we use the results of WIPPF and the balance model as resources. **8**

The next step is to help the partners tell their stories to the two therapists. The couple often comes to counceling polarized by power struggles that make them feel disconnected. In order to recreate safety and attachment, we use some resource oriented questions, for exampe the following “golden questions”: **9**

– How did you get to know each other? (Love, Trust, Tenderness, Time, Hope)

- In which situations during the last two months did you feel supported by your partner? (Reliability, Justice)
- In which situations during the last two months did you support your partner? (Reliability, Justice)
- Which little compliment did you make to your partner during the last two weeks? (Love, Politeness)
- Which little compliment did you get from your partner during the last two weeks? (Love, Politeness)
- What do you feel content or happy about in your relationship? (Hope, Contact)
- What does your partner feel content or happy about in your relationship? (Hope, Contact)
- If you think like your partner does, what is he/she proud of that you succeeded in together? (Meaning, Achievement)
- What do you think is the most important aspect in your relationship for your partner? (Trust, Honesty, Faithfulness)
- Which would be the best situation during the week to spend time together and talk to another? (Time, Contact)

These questions focus on the primary and secondary capabilities of the individual and the couple. Furthermore, they are helpful for recreating the feeling of a safe haven in their relationship, as this safe haven is a secure base for further development and differentiation. In individual development, as well as in the partnership situation everybody continually traverses different phases, which are characterized by the following three principles.

The stage of connectedness (attachment)

is based on the unborn child's dependence on her/his mother. It is loosened by a social symbiosis after the child's birth. The child is now dependent on the care and attention she/he gets from her/his social environment. She/he demands patience, time and attention and requires physical as well as social contact. For their part, the parents feel tied to the child through love, hope and responsibility. But the need for connectedness is something man feels his entire life.

The stage of differentiation

Differentiation is a basic principle of both physical and mental development. In socialization, the stage of differentiation is marked by the acquisition of socially desired behaviour. This happens in the differentiation of the person's ability to recognize and learn and in the formation of the secondary capabilities, which enable him to control nature and assert himself socially. At the same time, there is differentiation in one's ability to love. That is, we learn how and to whom we can reveal our feelings and in which social forms we can satisfy our urges. In other words, through differentiation our feelings take on a social shape. This process comes about through the confrontation with the structures that we find in our environment. **10**

The stage of detachment (autonomy)

Within the development of the individual, a specific unity can be achieved at each developmental level. Unity refers to the integration of the capabilities into an individual personality. Associated with it is an autonomy that takes on more and more importance until the individual reaches maturity. At the early stages of his development, a person is quite dependent in terms of connectedness, and even later on he needs to be guided by certain rules. But as he grows older, he needs this outside information of a lesser degree. He has adopted this information as concepts and makes his decisions with them in mind.

Detachment does not just mean that one turns away from an object or a person. The succession of detachment and connectedness makes it possible to establish contact with other persons and groups; that is, one can widen one's field of values and try new decisions, but perhaps also reevaluate old values. Many people swing back and forth between detachment and connectedness. They want to be independent but find they can't deal with their independence. Or they want the love and attention of a marriage partner but at the same time tend to evade it because of their desire for freedom.

In the next step of counceling the focus is on creating emotional responsiveness, raising the couple's acceptance of each other's experiences, creating new interactional situations and solutions for old problems.

Based on a safe bonding discussing problem and seeking their solutions will not harm anymore and a mature relationship is developing.

Tabatabai found that the following capabilities are connected to binational relationships: tolerance, empathy, openness, communication, integration of each other's values, self-awareness, acceptance, optimism and hope. **11**

Marriage and Partnership

Mulla Nasrudin (a Persian lay preacher) sat in the tea-room when a friend stormed in excitedly and wanted to speak to him. "I will marry, Mulla", his friend began, "and I am so excited. Mulla, have you yourself ever thought of marrying?"

Nasrudin answered: "Yes, I once thought of marrying. When I was young, I really wanted to get married. But I wanted the perfect woman. I went traveling, first to Damascus. I met a beautiful woman there that was graceful, friendly, and very spiritual but she didn't have any worldly knowledge.

I traveled on and came to Isfahan (a beautiful city of mosques in central Persia). There, I met a young woman that was spiritual and worldly, beautiful in many ways, but we weren't able to hold a conversation.

Ultimately, I went to Cairo and, there, I finally found her. She was of a profound spirituality, graceful, beautiful in every way, at home in this world and the worlds on the other sides. I knew I had found the perfect woman."

His friend wanted to know: "But you did not marry her, Mulla?" "No", Mulla Nasrudin said and shook his head, "she was waiting for the perfect man."

(according to Nossrat Peseschkian)

Summary

The satisfaction of partners in binational relationships seems to depend on the following aspects: is the couple childless or rearing children, supported by family or a social network? How does the environment react to the couple? An individual's ability to deal with stress and load and to better care for others/ children is strengthened by a couple's social support as well as securely bound partners. Securely bound partners are tuned in to each other like a mother to her baby. In Positive Psychotherapy, we support the clients' abilities to strengthen their bonding ability. Through this, primary and secondary capabilities are encouraged. A complementary approach is the theory of three stages of interaction. Both theories are based on the concepts of N. Peseschkian.

References

1 Van Mol C, de Valk H. 2014. Relationship satisfaction of European binational couples in the Netherlands. Working Paper 2014,13: 13

2 Van Mol C, de Valk H. (2014. Relationship satisfaction of European binational couples in the Netherlands. Working Paper 2014,13: 14

3 Master SL et al. 2009. A picture's worth- Partner photographs reduce experimentally induced pain. UCLA Department of Psychology. Los Angeles

4 Johnson S, Zuccarini D. 2009. Integrating sex and attachment in emotionally focused couple therapy. Journal of Marital&Family Therapy. Ottawa

5 Henrichs Ch. 2012. Psychodynamic Positive Psychotherapy emphasizes the Impact of Culture in the Time of Globalization. Psychology 3: 1148–1152

6 Peseschkian N. 1980, 1986. Positive Family Therapy: 179ff. Fischer. Frankfurt

7 Peseschkian N. 1980, 1986. Positive Family Therapy: 183–185. Fischer, Frankfurt

8 Remmers A. 1995, 2009. Wiesbaden Inventory for Positive Psychotherapy and Family Therapy WIPPF 2.0 International Version

9 Gesmann M, Rave Th. 2013 modified after Kindl-Beilfuß C. 2008, 2010. Fragen können wie Küsse schmecken. Carl-Auer. Heidelberg

10 Peseschkian N. 1980, 1986. Positive Family Therapy: 131–135. Fischer. Frankfurt

11 Tabatabai M. 2011. Ressourcen und Konfliktpotentiale in binationalen Partnerschaften. Tectum-Verlag. Marburg

Short CV

Mechthild Gesmann, MD
Specialist Internal Medicine (1996),
Psychosomatic Medicine and Psychotherapy (2004),
Senior physician at a Hospital for Psychosomatic Medicine,
Lecturer and Supervisor (Psychodynamic Psychotherapy and Positive Psychotherapy),
Since 2011 leading the Westfalian Institute for Positive Psychotherapie and Counceling, Bad Salzuflen, WIPPB

Psychoeducation Cultural Competencies (PCC)

Iwona Schimanski

The most common difficulties psychotherapists encounter in working with patients coming from different cultures are first and foremost the language barrier and a therapist's contact with foreignness in relation to accepted social norms and values held by Immigrant Patients (cf. Gavranidou 2008). These difficulties often lead to incorrect interpretation of emotions and thoughts expressed by Immigrant Patients or to overinterpretation of their behaviours. This phenomenon usually has a negative influence on the development of a therapeutic relationship. This is when a psychotherapist can feel helpless or irritated, whereas an Immigrant Patient can feel he/she is misunderstood or ignored (Ibid. 2008). Such misunderstandings lead to stagnation and resistance during therapy, which results in unsuccessful inpatient treatment.

Another problem in treating Immigrant Patients is a limited number of psychotherapists who have transcultural competencies or speak the target patients' native language, but also a limited number of so-called professional cultural interpreters (cf. Kluge 2015). Due to financial or logistic reasons, the above mentioned barriers are often ignored in clinical and psychotherapeutic practice.

Theoretical background of Psychoeducation Cultural Competencies (PCC)

Due to the mentioned difficulties and limitations in clinical and psychotherapeutic practice, the so-called Psychoeducation Cultural Competencies

(PCC) was introduced for Immigrant Patients at the Dr. Römer Clinic in Calw-Hirsau. The clinic deals with treating patients who suffer from mental and psychosomatic disorders. Most of them are immigrant patients from former Yugoslavia, Russia, Turkey, Poland, Italy, Spain and Portugal.

PCC is based on the Hyman concept of a "reference group" (1960) as a theoretical background. According to this concept, every person who joins a specific social group starts adapting his/her social categories, i.e. system of values, social norms and behaviour patterns to the social categories of this reference group. Numerous studies (e.g. Converse 1994; Ryan 2010; Merton & Kitt 1997 et al.) show how adapting to a group can lead to a change of one's social perception and worldview, but also to the so-called anomie, which arises from a feeling of alienation and purposelessness caused by sudden social changes and the collapse of the social structure (Merton 1938).

The phenomenon of adapting to a "reference group" resembles acculturation process, in other words, a cultural shock. As a result of a relatively long and intense influence of culture, every Immigrant is undergoing changes in psychological functioning. These changes usually take place due to an unconscious and automatically forced adaptation process, which initiates new social categories of different degree of adaptation (Berry 2003, p. 19). Thus, acculturation process is intense, requires a lot of mental effort and causes acute stress reactions. As is well known, stress (as cited in: Lazarus & Folkman 1987) can contribute to increased risk of mental problems (e.g. chronic neurotic, somatic, affective, schizotypal and other personality disorders) – as a result of incorrect cognitive interpretation of coping with this difficult situation (here: immigration) and the lack of appropriate regulating processes. Immigrant Patients usually do not associate their mental problems with adaptation processes and often ignore or repress them because of being ashamed.

The main psychotherapeutic instrument PCC used was the cognitive model by Judith S. Beck (2013), which is based on identifying situations that cause mental stress and the resulting strong emotional and behavioural reactions, and also automatic thoughts disturbing mental balance. Automatic thoughts usually depend on a situation and fulfil the function of the so-called "first" cognitive process. Most often, during such situations both intermediate beliefs, among others, general worldview and rules of conduct, and core beliefs, which do not depend on a situation, are updated; they are fixed and dogmatic. Most often, these beliefs are updated during a mental crisis and when combined with dysfunctional cognitive processes, they can lead to a mental disease. In the above mentioned project it was assumed that the acculturation process could be subject to continuous update of intrapsychic conflict between intermediate beliefs and automatic thoughts.

The development and objective of PCC

Taking into consideration the above mentioned difficulties and limitations in clinical and therapeutic practice with Immigrant Patients and using theoretical issues regarding understanding acculturation processes, a psychoeducational project for Immigrant Patients was developed. Its main objective was to present the most essential issues associated with the acculturation process and the resulting mental strains. The project lasted from April 2014 to May 2015 and brought together Immigrant Patients living in Germany for a short time and for a few years. The one thing the so-called heterogeneous group had in common was different nationality but the same way of communication, i.e. speaking – advanced or less advanced – German. In addition, it was an open group, which means new Immigrant Patients could join it at any time, yet, the maximum number of people allowed in the group was 12. The meetings were held once a week and lasted 50 minutes. The project put emphasis first and foremost on emotional and cognitive looking into key problems associated with acculturation stress, which contributes to both mental and behavioural disorders, among others, affective disorders, including intermediate factors evoking, e.g. a feeling of shame or low self-esteem; somatisation; isolation and avoidant tendency or schizoaffective disorders (repressing negative emotions), etc. (cf. Assion et al. 2009; Machleidt & Calliess 2005; Mokhtari Nejad et al. 2014; Kripper & Biligin 2009; Pflanz 1969; Zeiler & Zarifoglu 1997 et al.).

The main psychotherapeutic tool PCC used was the above mentioned cognitive model by Judith S. Beck (2013),

PCC topics

PCC were periodic topic-based meetings consisting in discussions in a group moderated by a psychotherapist or psychologist qualified in cognitive behavioural therapy. Apart from basic topic-related information, every meeting was supported by an exercise, which came in the form of a discussion. All thoughts, emotions, views, attitudes, etc. were written down on a flip chart. The topics of the meetings were as follows:

1. *Psychological acculturation and cultural adaptation strategies*
2. *Language function*
3. *Cultural differences in relation to the family model and the advantages of these differences*
4. *Self-stereotypization (cognitive errors on the example of the word "Foreigner")*
5. *Acculturation stages and crisis situations*

PCC meetings

Meeting 1: Psychological acculturation and cultural adaptation strategies

Immigrant Patients learned about the acculturation process (cultural adaptation process) and forms of cultural adaptation. They were also informed when one could speak about integration in general. At the beginning of the meeting, the concept of acculturation was defined and the main cultural strategies proposed by J. Berry (1990) were presented, i.e. the strategies of integration, separation, assimilation and marginalisation. Immigrant Patients became acquainted with the psychological function of adapting particular cultural strategies and the related discrepancies on the emotional, cognitive and behavioural level. Using their imaginations (*Imagine you are integrated/separated/assimilated…*), they were asked about automatic thoughts and emotions particular cultural strategies can cause. This is when Immigrant Patients realised cultural strategies could influence their lifestyle and self-development. During the meetings, one could experience a lot of wrong beliefs held by Immigrant Patients, e.g. their understanding of the concept of integration and being "integrated" with a new culture. This "feeling" was often identified with the length of time spent living abroad as immigrants.

Meeting 2: Language function

Immigrant Patients learned about language functions and its essential connotations with formulating and expressing thoughts. Immigrant Patients were made aware of how important knowledge of the host culture language was and what emotional and cognitive consequences they could encounter if they lacked this knowledge. At the beginning of the meeting, the role of language was defined and important language functions were suggested (referring to the concept of Sapir-Whorf and Piaget; in: Berry 1990) (e.g. *"Language is a transmitter of views and ideas", "Language transmits how a person behaves and reacts in different situations", "You can express your personality through language"*, etc.). During the meeting, consequences of the inability to speak the language were also discussed, i.e. abnormal reactions in stressful situations and unfavourable emotions, among others, fearful reactions (avoidance), shame and commonly experienced embarrassment in interpersonal relationships. Immigrant Patients often said they experienced strong emotions just because of the language, from bitterness and regret, through sadness or *"being under constant pressure"*, to anger toward themselves or sometimes to others. These emotions very often contribute to fear of coming in contact with others, becoming withdrawn or "conscious" isolation from others. Discussing this topic in the group and looking into most common thought mistakes (e.g. *"I'm stupid because I don't speak German"*) aimed at cognitive reformulation of unfavourable automatic thoughts, overcoming their inner barriers and motivating them to freely use German in a given social group.

Meeting 3: Cultural differences in relation to the family model and the advantages of these differences

Immigrant Patients learned about differences in relation to the family model and various characteristics from the perspective of collective and individual culture (on the basis of Hofstede 1987; Hofstede & Hofstede 2007). It was assumed that those discrepancies contributed to wrong interpretations and a selective way of noticing differences, and later to negative beliefs and prejudices among Immigrant Patients – in relation to parenting methods in the host culture. During the meetings, it was possible to notice clear contrasts in perceiving the family model, e.g. regardless of the length of stay in the host culture, Immigrant Patients unconsciously maintain and cultivate the parenting style they have been familiar with since they were "born". The meetings consisted of discussions about the most essential sources which influence maintaining one's "own" family model. The most common ones were language difficulties and choosing a separation lifestyle. Immigrant Patients realised those two sources favoured developing and consolidating wrong beliefs in relation to parenting methods in the host culture and maintaining the family model they are familiar with. This knowledge allowed them to better understand family conflicts: Patients as parents and their children born in the host culture or children who immigrated with them. Discussing this topic in the group and presenting the differences familiarised them with the source of conflicts and motivated them to draw possible benefits from the two cultures.

Meeting 4: Self-stereotypization (cognitive errors on the example of the word "Foreigner")

With the words "foreigner" and "tourist" in mind, Immigrant Patients realised their meanings first and foremost on the emotional and cognitive level. On the example of a sharp contrast, they were made aware of strong emotions and cognitive errors the word "foreigner" was associated with and its influence on a sense of belonging to the reference group, i.e. majority culture (compare "reference group" by Hyman). At the beginning of the meeting, Immigrant Patients were introduced with the linguistic meaning of the words "foreigner" and "tourist" ("foreigner", from the Latin word "peregrinus", refers to a person who comes from another country; "tourist" refers, among others, to a person who visits other countries). Then, they were asked questions about their associations and first and foremost about their automatic thoughts and the accompanying emotions connected with the above mentioned words. During the meetings, a lot of dysfunctional cognitive errors appeared, e.g. common statements included: *"A foreigner is a third-class person", "As foreigners, we are not welcome here", "One is a forever foreigner"*, etc. The accompanying emotions were very intense, sometimes even dramatic, e.g. *"As a foreigner, I feel humiliated all the time", "As a foreigner, I feel unwanted and misunderstood", "As a foreigner, I feel emptiness, I don't belong to any country"*, etc. Discussions in the group and presenting emotional and cognitive differences most often led to cognitive reformulating of unfavourable automatic thoughts and the accompanying intense emotions, and first and foremost to reducing inner tension.

Meeting 5: Acculturation stages and crisis situations

Immigrant Patients learned about different acculturation stages as exemplified by the concept of the "U-curve" by Lysgaard (Boski, 2009). The length and intensity of the acculturation process contributes to many changes at the psychological functioning level. Immigrant Patients were asked about their attitudes, mental attitudes and emotions – taking into consideration their immigration at the beginning and now. Crisis situations and mental load were also discussed. During the meetings, one could see the change of emotions over the years spent living as immigrants. These feelings were most often perceived as "Here and Now" and were very intense. One discussed also a constant feeling of "survival" that Immigrant Patients must face almost every day. Discussing this topic in the group led to better identification and verification of their inner changes at the emotional and cognitive level, which related to the degree of being adapted to the culture. Immigrant Patients realised mental attitude and cognitive errors played an important role in a sense of belonging to the group.

What do we learn about Immigrant Patients within the PCC project?

The example of the above mentioned meetings shows an Immigrant Patient as a person who, as a result of lack of a sense of belonging to majority culture, lives in constant inner tension, has a low self-esteem and is over sensitive to being constantly treated as a “foreigner”. It shows an Immigrant Patient who feels unaccepted and undervalued; whose feeling of shame is notoriously activated in situations beyond his/her control; who does not trust his/her skills and qualifications. Statements like *“I’m stupid because I speak with a foreign accent”*, *“I feel I don’t belong to them”* (*“to them”* meaning the Germans), *“I always have to prove that I also can, that I am also a human being”* appeared at the meetings. Such automatic thoughts and the accompanying negative emotions contribute to the fact that Immigrant Patients consciously withdraw from the majority culture, keep in touch with their cultural group and avoid conflicts for fear of making a mistake.

Summary

The project did not include evaluation studies, which would tell us what influence PCC had on mental improvement and increased motivation in stationary treatment among Immigrant Patients. Nevertheless, every meeting was documented, i.e. all statements and emotions written down on the flip chart were archived.

The main advantage of PCC consisted in bringing together Immigrant Patients of different origin in one group. They could realise that the difficulties connected with immigration did not concern only one culture but every Immigrant living in a foreign country, thanks to which Immigrant Patients experienced a certain form of “belonging to the group”, being the so-called “reference group”. Thus, they had a sense of belonging to the so-called “multicultural majority” and fully accepted diversity, which resulted in decreased intensity of expressed emotions. This effect was positively reflected in stationary treatment, i.e. Immigrant Patients more quickly entered into a therapeutic relationship during individual psychotherapeutic meetings, overcame their inner resistance and complexes connected, e.g. with the language, and were more willing to open up to contacts with other patients at the clinic. Through PCC, Immigrant Patients also received unconditional social support, which motivated them to overcome their inner resistance connected with their constant feeling of being “foreigners”. In addition, PCC enabled Immigrant Patients first and foremost to increase their awareness associated with acculturation difficulties.

Moreover, reporting the above mentioned meetings to doctors and other therapists increased their sensitiveness in contacts with Immigrant Patients and enabled them to better understand the main symptoms of their mental disease.

Summing up, one can say that PCC was a huge social support, which helped some Immigrant Patients achieve mental stability and inner motivation in stationary treatment.

References

Assion H.-J., Weiss A. & Korwischka J. 2009. Schizophrenie – ethnopsychiatrische und ethnopharmakologische Aspekte. Die Psychiatrie – Grundlagen und Perspektiven. Heft 1: 31–35.

Beck J. S. 2013. Praxis der Kognitiven Verhaltenstherapie. 2. Auflage. Wenheim: Beltz.

Berry J.W. (1990) Psychology of acculturation. Understanding individuals moving between cultures. In: Brislin RW (Hrsg.) Applied cross-cultural psychology London: Sage Publications: 232–253.

Berry J.W. 2003. Conceptual approaches to acculturation. In: Chun K.W., Organista P.M., Martin G. (Hrsg.). Acculturation, Advances in theory, measurement, and applied research. Washington: APA.

Boski P. 2009. Kulturowe ramy zachowań. Podręcznik psychologii międzykulturowej. Warschau: PWN und ACADEMICA.

Converse P.E. 1994. Theodore Mead Newcomb 1903–1984. A Biographical Memoir. Washington: National Academy of Sciences.

Gavranidou M. 2008. Besonderheiten von Psychotherapie bei Menschen mit Migrationshintergrund. PTK.

Hofstede G. 1983. National cultures in four dimensions. International Studies of Management & Organization: 13, 1/2: 46–74.

Hofstede G., Hofstede G.J. 2007. Kultury i organizacje. Zaprogramowanie umysłu. Wyd. II. Warszawa: Polskie Wydawnictwo Ekonomiczne.

Hyman H. 1960. Reflections on Reference Group. Public Opinion Quarterly 24,3: 383–396.

Kluge U. 2015. The (In)visible Third Person – Interpreters as language and cultural Interprets in psychosocial and psychotherapeutic services. Presentation during the First International Conference on Transcultural Psychiatry in Central European Countries in Gdynia (Poland).

Kripper M. & Biligin Y. 2009. Migration und Gesundheit. Berlin: Konrad Adenauer Stiftung: 54–55.

Lazarus R.S., Folkman S. 1987. Transactional theory and research on emotions and coping. European Journal of Personality. 1: 141–169.

Machleidt W. & Calliess I. T. 2005. Transkulturelle Psychiatrie und Migration – Psychische Erkrankungen aus ethnischer Sicht. In: Die Psychiatrie – Grundlagen und Perspektiven. Heft 2: 77–84.

Merton R.K. 1938. Social Structure and Anomie. American Sociological Review. 3,5: 672–682.

Merton R.K., Kitt A.S. 1997. Contributions to the Theory of Reference Group Behavior. Classical Tradition in Psychology: The American Tradition. 3: 129–153.

Mokhtari Nejad R., Eser-Valeri D., Falkai P. 2014. Psychische Erkrankungen und Migration – es ist nicht so, wie es erscheint. Die Psychiatrie – Grundlagen und Perspektiven. Heft 1: 56–60

Pflanz M. 1969. Soziokulturelle Faktoren und psychische Störungen. Fortschritte der Neurologie und Psychiatrie. Grenzgeb. 28: 471–508.

Ryan J.W. 2010. Samuel A. Souffer and the American Soldier. Journal of Historical Biography. 7: 100–137.

Zeiler J. & Zarifoglu Fuat. 1997. Psychische Störungen bei Migranten: Behandlung und Prävention. Zeitschrift für Sozialreform. 4: 300–334.

Short CV

Iwona Schimanski, PhD in Clinical Psychology with the main emphasis on cultural Psychiatry and Psychotherapy, iwona@schimanski.name

Expirience of distance consultation of children and adolescents with disabilities

I.E. Kupriyanova, B.A. Dashiyeva, I.S. Karaush

The article presents the experience of remote consultation of children with disabilities living in rural or remote areas with lack of access to specialized services in connection with disabling illness and family circumstances. The organization of the stages of counseling, which allocate the groups of children depending on the amount of necessary aid has been described. The advantage of the proposed form of counseling is to identify the borderline mental disorders and behavioral disorders at an early stage, the possibility of timely psychotherapy/ psycho-pharmacological correction and prevention. The socioeconomic importance of this technology was marked.

Keywords: remote consultation, children with disabilities, psychological rehabilitation

ZAGADNIENIE KONSULTACJI NA ODLEGLOść DZIECI Z OGRANICZENIAMI ZDROWOTNYMI

I.J. Kuprijanowa, B.A.Daszijewa, I.S.Karausz

Instytut Zdrowia Psychycznego, Tomsk, Rosja

W referacie przedstawione zostało zagadnienie konsultacji na odległość dzieci z ograniczeniami zdrowotnymi, zamieszkującymi tereny wiejskie lub oddalone od dużych skupisk miejskich. Miejsca te charakteryzują się niepełnym dostępem do specjalistycznych usług w zakresie indywidualnej opieki zdrowotnej osób niepełnosprawnych oraz trudnymi warunkami rodzinnymi. W materiale opisana została organizacja etapów konsultacji, pozwalająca na wydzielenie grup dzieci w zależności od zakresu potrzebnej pomocy. Korzyścią omawianej formy poradnictwa jest rozpoznanie zaburzeń psychicznych i behawioralnych na wczesnym etapie, możliwość zastosowania terminowej psychoterapii/psychofarmakologicznego leczenia oraz podjęcie odpowiednich działań prewencyjnych. W referacie podkreślone zostało także socialno-ekonomiczne znaczenie opisanej techniki.

Słowa kluczowe: konsultacje na odległość, dzieci z ograniczeniami zdrowotnymi, rehabilitacja psychologiczna

The trend of modernity in the rehabilitation of children with disabilities is to promote the creation of various services using innovative technologies to meet the needs of children and contributing to the active position of the family in overcoming the limitations imposed by the disability (Raina P. et al., 2004; W. Simpson et al., 2010; Simşek, I. E. et al., 2014). The essential point is the revision of the rehabilitation paradigm from a predominantly medical rehabilitation to psychotherapeutic methods, socio-psychological, psycho-pedagogical impact on disabled children and their social environment (Koren', E. V., 2011). Such features of Russia as a large area with low population density, limiting the availability of specialized care in remote areas, economic problems, determine the need for new forms of assistance. One of the vulnerable groups is children and adolescents with disabilities.

Activities, services and systems associated with health practiced remotely through information and communication technology for management and research in the field of health protection previously were determined as "tele-health" (World Health Organization, 1997), currently the term "tele-"is deprecated and replaced by the concept of "e-health" or "remote consultation". It includes the transmission and the storage of data for the diagnosis, the monitoring and the accounting (World Health Organization, 2010).

There is evidence of the effectiveness of the use of psychotherapy by remote method in the treatment of the social phobia, the generalized anxiety disorder and other anxiety disorders (B. T. Tulbure, Månsson, K. N., G. Andersson, 2012; Kirkpatrick, T., L. Manoukian, Dear B. F., Johnston L., Titov, N., 2013), depression (Dear BF, et al., Aust N Z Psych, 2013). It is also reported about the application of this method in children and adults with the neurological disorders, the speech disorders and the autism spectrum disorders (A. Hill, Theodoros D., 2002; Mashima, P. A., C. R. Doarn, 2011; E. Whitehead, Dorfman V. et all., 2012; P. L. Pearl, Sable, C. et all.,

2014). The aid system with the use of the distance technologies can be cost-effective, because it does not require large additional costs, but rather redistributes existing resources (B. Grady, 2012 R. Thara, Sujit J., 2013).

The provision of telemedicine services may cover not only the residents of rural or remote areas, also the urban residents who have difficulties with access to the specialist services due to disability, family difficulties and problems with transport (Theodoros D. G. 2008, 2012). It appears to be a promising application of such methods in children and adolescents with disabilities, especially in terms of distance or home study. Today for children the information technologies are a part of everyday life (learning, playing and communication), so this method of service is perceived positively (J. C. Coleman, L. Hendry, 1999; Holtz, P., M. Appel, 2011). In addition, it has been suggested that this technology allows to take into account socio-cultural and ethno-cultural values of the family and to ensure public support (E. Lalor, M. Brown, E. Cranfield, 2000; Myers C., 2005). We conducted a study of the mental health of various categories of children and adolescents related to "children with disabilities: intellectual, speech problems, cerebral palsy, hearing impairments, somatic diseases.

In this article we present the experience of remote consultation of children with abnormal development and being home schooled as a fragment of the study of mental health of children with disabilities. As a rule, this category of children is out of the attention of specialists of psychological and psychotherapeutic services.

Materials:

Schoolchildren of special schools (Tomsk region) and school of social adaptation of disabled children (Ulan-Ude city of the Republic of Buryatia), who are learning home/distance in rural or remote areas with limited access to specialized services in connection with the peculiarities of disabling illness, family circumstances and problems with transport.

The inclusion criteria in the group of remote consultations in these category children were:

- Mental disorders and disorders requiring systematic follow-up and therapy.
- Violations of socio-psychological adaptation

- Psychological problems associated with the primary disease and the stages of development
- Impaired parent-child relationship
- Stay in the conditions of difficult situations

The target audience, which, in our opinion, it is expedient to conduct remote consultation, are the parents of children this category. An important aspect of this problem is a fear of stigma among family members of children with disabilities, which manifests itself in a closed family system and the avoidance of care, even when the possibility of it's receiving (Kupriyanova I.E., Dashieva B.A., Karaush I.S., 2014). Often in such families, the psychological difficulties a child with disabling illness and development are ignored.

One-third of parents (32–35%) are showing low level of parental competence of the child's illness and the lack of motivation to obtain information on this subject. In their view, the rehabilitation is a business of professionals; such parents exhibit the rental installation, delegating responsibility for the health and ensuring the psychological and educational needs of the child's medical, public and government institutions. Almost 50% of the interviewed parents show interest, but they use biased, unreliable information, which is reflected in their actions in the rehabilitation process. Only 15–18% of parents is open to information, new data, and participates actively in rehabilitation activities, collaborating with doctors, teachers and psychologists. It is worth noting the presence of conjugated linkages between parent's rehabilitation strategies and their level of education. Also the remote consultation was conducted with teachers, psychologists, health workers of the correctional schools, working with children with disabilities. In the psychological support of children with special needs in terms of special schools we found a lack of competent adults working with children with disabilities in relation to psychological, personality characteristics of children with developmental disabilities that promotes intolerance towards them (Kupriyanova I.E., Dashieva B.A., Karaush I.S., 2013). This was manifested in the labeling, inadequate and inappropriate expectations of requirements, thus created the risk of violations of adaptation of the schoolchildren, neurotic, affective reactions and behavioral disorders.

The use of distance counseling is contraindicated in the presence of the child's manifestations of mental disorders requiring hospital treatment; severe intellectual impairment (mental retardation moderate, severe stage); exacerbation of chronic or acute somatic pathology; the refusal of the parents of the child or the child from the survey, in the absence of technical capacity for the implementation of the technology. Logistical support includes the availability of the premises, equipped with a computer with Internet connection, a webcam and installed Scype.

Prerequisites for the effectiveness of remote consultations are: a compliance with the law on personal data protection; a compliance with ethics Committee requirements for studies of this kind (the informed consent of parents of children with disabilities and adolescents over the age of 14 years, the observance of ethical standards); a compliance with the rehabilitation interventions standards of medical care

In the implementation of the consultation highlighted the following stages:

1. The organizational stage (selection of the target group in accordance with the indications for the distance technology and organizational issues – an informed consent, the technical equipment).
2. Information-preparatory stage: screening of parents and teachers; the analysis of personnel files.
3. The Advisory stage (consultations)
4. The formation of the conclusions and the forecast, the determination of rehabilitation strategies.

At the organizational stage have been determined the number of school children studying at home schooling; teachers and parents were provided with information about remote counseling, forms of conduct and the necessary technical requirements.

In special schools, where the study was conducted, 550 pupils have been studied. including 112 home learning pupils. 35 parents/guardians of children have decided to consult on-line.

On information-preparatory stage, parents and teachers were asked specially designed questionnaires to identify "problem areas". The medical records, hospital records and personnel files were studied. The information from the class teachers, psychologists, social workers about difficulties of particular pupil has been collected. This helped to navigate in the characteristics of the studied contingent, to assume existing child and his entourage resources. The result is a dedicated group of 15 schoolchildren 10–14 years old who need the priority assistance. The reasons of home or distance learning were cerebral palsy, neurological pathology, trauma, post-operative state. These conditions were combined with hearing loss (sensorineural hearing loss III-IVñòåïåíè), psychological disorders and speech development. In 53.3% of cases (8 pupils)

At the consultative stage, the counseling of children and parents in remote conditions with the use of necessary equipment was conducted. Forms of distance counseling:
- One-time consultation;
- Episodic counseling (upon request);
- Surveillance for a long period of time (academic year).

The duration of treatment and frequency of sessions was determined by the actual condition of child, his motivation for this type of assistance and attitude of parents.

During the primary counseling session, the collecting objective and subjective anamnesis was conducted; the complaints, the content of difficulties, previous treatment were revealed. The adaptations to the learning environment, the level of social adaptation (relationships with peers, the ability to solve interpersonal problems), personality traits (self-esteem, level of aspiration and aspiration for self-development) were studied. To clarify the clinical data, if necessary, were used the scale and questionnaires (scales anxiety CMAS, depression scale M. Kovac, questionnaire on the identification of suicide risk, assessment of coping behavior).

The single consultative session was held to three schoolchildren. The consultations addressed the issues related to psychological difficulties in the interpersonal relations; the help in identifying personality characteristics in order to optimize the professional orientation; the teaching methods remove anxiety and the tension in stressful situations (before medical intervention). In the occasional advice needed 7 pupils. The range of problems included issues with the ongoing divorce of parents; the change of residence and the adaptation to a new team; adaptation to training loads after a period of prolonged hospitalization; problems in interpersonal relationships (love); support of children and parents during the stay in a specialized inclusive summer camp. The surveillance for a long period was conducted with five students who had negative emotional reactions, mental maladjustment and suicidal behavior.

At the stage of forming conclusions and outlook, the analysis of data was conducted. It has allowed us to refer schoolchildren to the following groups depending on the volume and nature of aid.

- Group 1 – children without mental disorders and signs of mental distress, experiencing temporary psychological difficulties. In this case the information and psycho hygienic recommendations are sufficient.
- Group 2 – children with signs of mental distress, who can be attributed to the "risk group" for the development of mental disorders, with prolonged and/or intense psychological, emotional problems, having some symptoms insufficient for diagnosis of mental disorders. The psychotherapy, the correction of the parent-child relationship and the parent counseling with the aim of increasing parental competence was conducted.
- Group 3 – children with acute symptoms of mental disorders. Depending on the level of existing violations, the consultation was accompanied by the appointment of pharmacological therapy and supervision. Participants were also given recommendations for treatment in specialized medical institutions and conducting additional tests.

Moreover, may be given the recommendations:

- For treatment in specialized medical institutions
- Recommendations for survey methods
- Recommendations for referral to other health care professionals' profiles
- Recommendations for appeal to the social, law enforcement services, rehabilitation centers and public organizations working with disabled children.

A separate form of distance counseling is forwarding. The study of mental health of children with special needs in the regions of Siberia took place in the mode of expeditions conducted twice a year for four years. Remote consultation was used both at the initial organizational stage and between expeditions. At the organizational stage was coordinated by a number of participants, the surveys were conducted with parents and children predetermined objectives and areas of counseling. This preparatory work will allow reducing time and improving the efficiency of resource allocation. Between expeditions, the main objective was to provide dynamic monitoring of the children and feedback from parents and teachers. This form of organization provides remote consultations timeliness of care improves accessibility and promotes the growth of parental competence and responsibility for the rehabilitation process.

Conclusion

Remote consultation provides an opportunity to obtain access to specialized medical and psychological assistance to children with disabilities and their parents in terms of remote access, as well as in the forwarding mode for specialized assistance.

The use of distance counseling can improve the efficiency of rehabilitation of mental disorders in specific correctional school, reduce the risk of borderline mental disorders in children with disabilities, behavior disorders or to detect them early and timely start of therapy and/or corrective process. This form of counseling provides the competence of parents in the problems associated with disabling illness with their children, and reduces the level of stigmatization of families of children with disabilities. In terms of socioeconomic crisis, this form is timely and relevant.

References

Bower P., Gilbody S. Stepped care in psychological therapies: access, effectiveness, and efficiency: narrative literature review. Br J Psychiatry 2005; 186:11–17.

Coleman J.C., Hendry L. The nature of adolescence, ed 3. London, Routledge, 1999.

Grady B. Promises and limitations of telepsychiatry in rural adult mental health care. World Psychiatry 2012; 11:199–201.

Hill A., Theodoros D. Research into telehealth applications in speech-language pathology. J Telemed Telecare 2002; 8:187–196.

Holtz P., Appel M. Internet use and video gaming predict problem behavior in early adolescence. J Adolesc 2011; 34:49–58.

Kirkpatrick T., Manoukian L., Dear B.F., Johnston L., Titov N. A feasibility open trial of internet-delivered cognitive-behavioural therapy (iCBT) among consumers of a non-governmental mental health organisation with anxiety PeerJ. 2013; 1: e210.

Koren' E. V. Theoretical and methodological approaches to the study of integrated psychosocial rehabilitation in child psychiatry // Mental health issues of children and adolescents. 2011 (11). 2. P. 60–69.

Kupriyanova Irina Evgenyevna, Dashiyeva Bairma Antonovna, Karaush Irina Sergeevna Mental Health State of Children with Disabilities and Principles of Rehabilitation. Pediatrics Research International Journal, Vol. 2014 (2014), Article ID 149505, DOI: 10.5171/2014.149505

Kupriyanova I.E., Dashieva B.A., Karaush I.S. Quality of life and mental health of teachers working in different education systems (general, correctional, inclusive). TSPU Bulletin. – 11 (139) – 2013. P. 87–93.

Lalor E., Brown M., Cranfield E. Telemedicine: its role in speech and language management for rural and remote patients. ACQ Speech Pathol Aus 2000; 2:54–55.

Mashima P.A., Doarn C.R. Overview of telehealth activities in speech-language pathology. Telemed e-Health 2008; 14:1101–1117.

Myers C. Telehealth applications in head and neck oncology. J Speech Lang Pathol Audiol 2005; 29: 125–129.

Pearl P.L., Sable C., Evans S., Knight J., Cunningham P., Lotrecchiano G.R., Gropman A., Stuart S., Glass P., Conway A., Ramadan I., Paiva T., Batshaw M.L., Packer R.J. International Telemedicine Consultations for Neurodevelopmental Disabilities. Telemed J E Health. 2014 Mar 24.

Raina P., O'Donnell M., Schwellnus H., Rosenbaum P., King G., Brehaut J., Russell D., Swinton M., King S., Wong M., Walter S. D., Wood E. Caregiving process and caregiver burden: conceptual models to guide research and practice // BMC Pediatr. 2004. 4,4. 13 pages, http://www.biomedcentral.com/1471--2431/4/1

Simpson W., Cowie L., Wilkinson L., Lock N., Monteith G. The Effectiveness of a Community Intensive Therapy Team on Young People's Mental Health Outcomes // Child and Adolescent Mental Health. 2010. Vol. 15. 4. P. 217–223.

Simşek I. E., Erel S., Simşek T. T., Atasavun Uysal S., Yakut H., Yakut Y., Uygur F. Factors related to the impact of chronically disabled children on their families // Pediatr Neurol. 2014. 50 (3). Đ. 255–261.

Thara R., Sujit J. //World Psychiatry 2013; 2: 80

Theodoros D.G. Telerehabilitation for service delivery in speech-language pathology. J Telemed Telecare 2008; 14:221–224.

Theodoros D.G. A new era in speech-language pathology practice: innovation and diversification. Int J Speech Lang Pathol 2012; 14:189–199.

Tulbure B.T., Månsson K.N., Andersson G. Internet treatment for social anxiety disorder in Romania: study protocol for a randomized controlled trial Trials. 2012, 13:202.

Whitehead E., Dorfman V., Tremper G., Kramer A., Sigler A., Gosman A. Telemedicine as a means of effective speech evaluation for patients with cleft palate. Ann Plast Surg. 2012, 68(4):415–417.

World Health Organization: A health telematics policy in support of WHO's Health-for-All Strategy for global health development. Report of the WHO group consultation on health telematics, 11–16 December, Geneva, 1997. http://whqlibdoc.who.int/hq/1998/WHO_DGO_98.1.pdf.

2World Health Organization: Telemedicine: opportunities and developments in Member States. Report on the second global survey on eHealth, 2010. http: //www.who.int/goe/publications/goe_telemedicine_2010.pdf

Short CV

Kupriyanova Irina Evgenyevna, doctor of medical Sciences, Professor, Mental Health Research Institute "; Tomsk, Russia. redo@mail.tomsknet.ru

Dashieva Bairma Anatolievna, candidate of medical Sciences, senior researcher of the Mental Health Research Institute "; Tomsk, Russia. bairma2009@mail.ru

Karaush Irina Sergeevna, candidate of medical Sciences, senior researcher of the Mental Health Research Institute "; Tomsk, Russia.anir7@yandex.ru.

Therapeutic Housing Community: Social Psychiatry in the Treatment and Integration of Traumatized Female Refugees

Malgorzata Symonowicz

The article is an extended version of the presentation at the First International Conference on Transcultural Psychiatry in Central European Countries, on 24–26.04.2015 in Gdynia, Poland.

The Supervised Housing Community Project for Female Migrants is one of the projects within the Berlin Center for Torture Victims, established in 1992 to treat victims of torture and war-time violence. The Berlin Center for Torture Victims treats and cares for around 400 patients each year from about 40 different countries. They receive both medical and psychotherapeutic help as well as social assistance. Other departments of the Center are the various out-patient sections for adults, children and adolescents as well as the Day Clinic.

In the following I will concentrate on the Supervised Housing Community Project and illustrate how the social psychiatry approach can be adapted to the treatment of traumatized refugees.

The Supervised Housing Community Project

The Supervised Housing Community for Female Migrants has been operating since 2007 and it is already well-known to many professionals working with refugees in Berlin. Women are referred to the project by those professionals or come on recommendation of other clients and community members. The participation in our project is voluntary. The pre-requisite for admission is the functional impairment caused by the mental disease persisting over six months.

The project is one of the numerous care providers within the Berlin community mental healthcare network. The multicultural and multilingual team includes social workers, social educational workers, psychologists and psychotherapists as well as interns and volunteers. Also we work together with physicians, psychiatrists, physiotherapist and numerous interpreters from the Centre for Torture Victims. Presently (June 2015) the project offers 45 places, including 4 places in the supervised shared apartment. The rest of our clients live at scattered sites, like refugee shelters, women's shelter or rented apartments. They are getting assistance and treatment at their homes and the facilities of the project.

The low participant-to-staff ratio enables a very intensive treatment. Each of the clients has one steady carer (*Betreuerin*), assisting her 4 to 12 hours weekly. As required, the individual psychotherapy takes place for 1 or 2 hours a week. The clients are in relation with at least 2 and mostly 3–4 cooperating team-members from different occupational groups. Due to the clients' gender-specific violence experience only women are working with them.

The project offers long-term treatment: clients participate in the program for one year or more, on average 3 to 4 years. The duration is limited by the client's need of this type of professional help. The treatment consists of three phases. 1st settling in and establishing the working alliance, 2nd therapeutic phase with intensive participation in groups, 3rd starting to live independently. The general goals of the treatment are the psychosocial rehabilitation and participation in the society.

Our clients

All of our clients of the Supervised Housing Community Project are female, from the age of 18 onwards. They come from 15 different countries, most of them from Russia, Turkey, Afghanistan, Syria, Lebanon, Kosovo and Bosnia. The majority of the clients are Muslim. They have different educational backgrounds ranging from illiteracy to university degree and different occupational experience. Many of them are disabled. Their family situations vary. Although their socio-demographic characteristics differ, they all share the experience of violence, like exposure to war, imprisonment and torture, or human trafficking. Many of them have witnessed relatives and friends being tortured and killed. Currently they have well founded worries about family members and friends left behind. They have been through a long and dangerous journey to Germany. It is characteristic of our clients to have gender-specific violence experience, like rape, sexual harassment, domestic violence and all forms of gender based discrimination.

Post-migration living problems

After arriving in Germany our clients faced numerous problems, like difficult economic circumstances, poor housing situation, unemployment due to lack of work permission or their mental health problems, limited access to health services and – first of all – an insecure legal status. By the admission to the project many of the clients are applying for asylum and only a few are recognized refugees or have a resident permit for humanitarian reasons. Most of them do not speak German. They feel overwhelmed and isolated from the society. In many cases they are suffering from discrimination and xenophobia. The ongoing stress results in physical health problems.

Their partners, children and other family members are also affected by the past and present circumstances or – in many cases – mental disease. Those clients, who are domestic violence victims, often stay in a relationship with the perpetrators. Their own ethnic community has both protective and oppressive effects. On the one hand it gives them affiliation and support, on the other hand it makes them captives of their traditional roles and stigmatizes them because of their mental illness, and they are a "disgrace" to their families.

Legal status

The lack of a safe legal status is a huge burden in the treatment of our clients. First of all, persons without documents are not entitled to take part in the project. Then the long-lasting asylum procedure and the threat of the imminent deportation make our clients feel helpless and hopeless about the future. A temporary resident permit depending on the health status of the client creates a vicious circle in the therapy: as soon as the person gets well, she exposes herself to the risk of deportation. Numerous studies (for instance: Laban et al. 2004) confirm our observations that the long asylum procedure increases the health problems and has a negative impact on the treatment results.

Mental health disorders

The most common diagnosis among our clients are trauma-related disorders, predominantly post-traumatic stress disorder. Anxiety disorders, depressive disorders, somatoform disorder and adjustment disorder have high prevalence. Diagnosis of schizophrenia or alcohol dependency occurs rarely. The level of co-morbidity is very high. Many of the clients misuse psychopharmaca and other medication. Some of them have already had severe mental health problems before arriving to Germany, but only a few were in psychiatric treatment before.

The social psychiatry approach

The Supervised Housing Community Project is based on the social psychiatry approach, which draws from different scientific perspectives such as sociology, cultural anthropology, cultural and social psychology to outline the relevance of interpersonal and cultural factors for mental health (Morgan & Bhugra 2010).

Social psychiatry is concerned with the mutual effects of the social environment and the mental health of the individual. It emphasizes the influence of the socioeconomic circumstances and the adverse life events on the mental wellbeing (Morgan & Bhugra 2010). Accordingly, the social psychiatry approach concentrates on the client's psychosocial rehabilitation and facilitates the empowerment and the social inclusion of the persons with mental illness (Brückner 2010). The therapeutic interventions aim at re-establishing the client's resources and self-efficacy (Maier 2007).

Psychosocial rehabilitation

The basis of the treatment within the project is the working alliance between client and carer to promote the client's personal responsibility and to avoid patronizing her. By the admission most of our clients are not aware of the possibilities of the treatment-offers available in Germany. Giving them appropriate information on this is essential for establishing a safe and transparent setting. Client's resources, perceptions, expectations and jointly developed solutions to her problems forms the treatment- and rehabilitation plan. The "side-effect" of the plan scheduled for one year and different life-fields is drawing a perspective for the future, most of our traumatised clients are lacking in. Since the project is embedded in the community mental healthcare of the city of Berlin, the treatment plan is submitted to evaluation by the Social Psychiatry Services. The client takes part in the assessment procedure.

The treatment in the Housing Community Project does not focus on the client's prior traumatic experiences, but on her current problems related to post-migration stressors. The post migration living problems have a significant impact on the mental health of asylum seekers (Birck et al. 2002; Brandmaier 2011). According to Laban (Laban et al. 2014) the negative effect of the adverse life events after arrival in the host country can even exceed the influence of the events before migration. The therapeutic work through past trauma begins mostly after months of recovery, using elements of the cognitive behavioral or psychodynamic therapeutic approach.

The main fields of our work are improvement of the housing conditions, applying for financial assistance, access to education and to the job market, support by treatment of non-psychiatric diseases, and by obtaining a safe legal status. We deliver necessary information about living in the German society. Our volunteers are offering German classes, to improve the clients' language skills. We make home visits and various "out of the office" interventions, for example: training in the use of public transport, dealing with bureaucracy and accompanying clients to authorities, including all the nitty-gritty aspects of everyday life. We cooperate with and mediate between client and lawyers, refugee shelter-staff or landlords, teachers, medical specialists and other professionals and institutions. The aim of the interventions is to give our clients tools and skills for empowering them in their daily life.

The project is offering also a day-structure, filled with group- and free-time activities. Structuring time is particularly important for our clients due to their unemployment and social withdrawal. As we recognize the importance of social connections for mental health, we offer our clients opportunity to gain social and emotional support in the group.

Group activities concern psychoeducation about trauma, dialectical behaviour therapy (DBT) skills training, artistic expressions and physical exercise. The participation in the groups helps the clients in understanding their reactions and dealing with mental stress as well as shifting from complaints to resources. Sharing their difficult experience with the others results in the reduction of shame and feeling of guilt. The clients regain trust and acceptance among the others.

To break the social isolation and focus on positive emotions our clients take part in joint meals, outings in Berlin and summer trips outside the city. Some of the clients continue to meet even beyond the project. The families of the clients are also involved in the treatment in the form of psychoeducation about mental illness and, if necessary, mediation between family members.

'Client-tailored' treatment

The multiple traumatic experiences and the complex problems of the refugees hardly fit in with most psychotherapeutic approaches and methods. A treatment suitable for this group has to be comprehensive to include all aspects of the client's life. The social psychiatry approach enables a widely individualized, 'client-tailored' treatment, combining professional perspectives of different occupational groups.

Social inclusion and integration

Facilitating the social inclusion of people with mental health problems is major focus of social psychiatry. It is even a more pivotal issue for refugees with mental illness, facing multiple discrimination. The project aims to bridge the gap between the clients and the society. We are informing, translating, mediating, standing on our client's side to enhance her ability to act in the German society and facilitate the integration as the acculturation strategy resulting in the best outcomes with regard to mental health (Berry 1997).

Easy access to the treatment

To reach our target group the project must be easily accessible. Many of our clients are not entitled to get full medical treatment because of their legal status during the asylum procedure, but nevertheless we are allowed to include them in the project. The priority given to the psychosocial rehabilitation in the Supervised Housing Community helps the clients in overcoming their fear and distrust against psychiatry and psychotherapy. The informal and flexible role of the carer, different from the stereotypical doctor or therapist role, helps the clients to open up and involves them in the project.

Empowerment of the clients

The client's empowerment, defined as discovering strengths and competences of the person and encouraging her to take matters into her own hands (Brandmaier 2011), plays a crucial role in the social psychiatry approach. In the Supervised Housing Community, we encourage our clients to be active participants in their treatment and to regain control over their lives, a feeling that a traumatised person has lost. The transition between being patronized and being independent is extremely hard to most of our clients because of their experience of being discriminated against as a woman, migrant, minority-member, etc. Restoring the client's self-efficacy and self-esteem is especially important in coping with trauma (Maier 2007). In the therapeutic interventions we concentrate on establishing and strengthening of the client's resources as a tool of her empowerment.

Cultural competence in the treatment

Cultural competence is essential in our work. The team takes part in trainings, internal consultation and regular external supervision concerning culturally relevant issues such as culturally-based explanations of mental disorders, psychosomatic expression of illness and compliance in the pharmacotherapeutic treatment.

Beside the psychiatric diagnosis we use the level of the client's needs, difficulties and resources for assessment and evaluation of her progress in the treatment. It helps us in respecting the cultural context and individual concepts of mental recovery. An indispensable part of our work is the co-operation with the experienced interpreters from the Berlin Center for Torture Victims, bringing their language skills as well as knowledge about the client's culture.

Many of the team members are migrants or have a migrant background. The exact matching of our clients' cultural backgrounds is not intended, although in some cases it is effective in improving care for ethnic minority groups (Chow & Andermann 2009). Since the important goal of the treatment is the integration into the society, we encourage our clients to interact across ethnic lines and not to withdraw into their ethnic community.

Limitations of the social psychiatry approach

Although we notice many advantages from applying the social psychiatry approach in our work with traumatized refugee women, we encounter also its limitations.

The rehabilitation within the local community is the underlying idea of social psychiatry. Our clients have lost their original local communities and have not managed to find a place in the new one yet. Besides social withdrawal as one of the post-traumatic symptoms and the socioeconomic barriers, the integration into the community is limited by frequently moving house. Our clients, like other asylum seekers and refugees, have to move many times from one district to another, due to decisions of the social security department or difficulties in finding an affordable apartment in Berlin. The jurisdiction within the Social Psychiatry Services also changes because of the move. Building up a social network between the clients, within our project and cooperating organizations, turns out to be much easier than connecting them with the German society. Social networks limited to persons similar in their socio-demographic characteristics are unfortunately less useful for the migrants' mental health than more heterogeneous networks (Türkmen 2014).

On the basis of our experiences in integrating the clients into the existing mental health network we notice that their access to the community mental health services in Berlin is very limited. The community mental health services and other health care providers have not enough staff speaking the required languages and having the necessary cultural competences as well as relevant legal knowledge. Numerous studies confirm that migrants are under-represented in social psychiatry institutions as clients (Arslan et al. 1998; Basche & Kaouk 2003; Bezirk Mitte, OE Qalitätsentwicklung, Planung und Koordination 2011). While community mental health services do not create appropriate requirements for the treatment of traumatized refugees, the migrant-centered projects do not have sufficient capacities to cover the needs of this group.

Conclusion

The analysis of the treatment methods within the Supervised Housing Community shows a great usefulness of the social psychiatry approach in addressing the specific needs of traumatized refugees. Social psychiatry offers a flexible framework for dealing with their complex problems. It focuses on the client's current life situation, strengthens her resources and self-efficacy. Enhancing the client's integration and social participation is an important issue in this approach as well. Essential requirements for effective treatment of refugees are easy access, cultural competence and knowledge about specific legal issues the majority of the community mental health providers are lacking in. The Supervised Housing Community Project fills this gap and enables the traumatized refugees to benefit from the advantages of the social psychiatry approach.

References

Arslan S. Uslucan H.H. Flötotto Ch. 1998. Sozialpsychiatrische Versorgung von Migranten. In: Koch E. Özek M. Pfeiffer W.M. Schepker R. Chancen und Risiken von Migration. Deutsch-türkische Perspektiven. Freiburg: Lambertus: 52–62.

Basche J. Kaouk M. 2003. Qualitätssicherung durch niedrigschwellige kulturspezifische Hilfen –Möglichkeiten der Mobilisierung informeller Ressources am Beispiel der sozialpsychiatrischen Versorgung arabischer Familien. In: Borde T. David M (ed.) Gut Versorgt? Migrantinnen und Migranten im Gesundheits- und Sozialwesen. Frankfurt/M: Mabuse-Verlag: 203–223.

Berry J. W. 1997. Immigration, acculturation, and adaptation. Applied Psychology: An International Review, 46, 1: 5–34

Bezirk Mitte von Berlin, Bezirk Mitte, OE Qalitätsentwicklung, Planung und Koordination. 2011. Migration und Gesundheit im Bezirk Berlin Mitte. Gesundheitliche und soziale Lage der Bevölkerung unter Berücksichtigung des Migrationshintergrundes (Spezialbericht). Berlin: Bezirk Berlin Mitte.

Birck A. 2002. Folterüberlebende nach psychotherapeutischer Behandlung. Untersuchung ehemaliger Patienten zwei Jahre nach Therapieende. In A. Birck A. Pross C. Lansen J. (ed.) Das Unsagbare. Die Arbeit mit Traumatisierten im Behandlungszentrum für Folteropfer Berlin. Berlin: Springer: 227–238.

Brandmaier M. 2011. Wie gestaltet sich die Bewältigung traumatischer Erlebnisse im Exil? Möglichkeiten der psychosozialen Unterstützung traumatisierter Flüchtlinge in Deutschland, Berlin: LIT Verlag.

Brückner B. 2010. Geschichte der Psychiatrie. Bonn: Psychiatrie Verlag.

Chow W, Andermann L. 2009. ACT Tailored for Ethnocultural Communities of Metropolitan Toronto, Psychiatric Services. A Journal of the American Psychiatric Association, 60(4): 847.

Laban C.J. Gernaat H.B.P.E. Komproe I.H. Schreuders G.A. De Jong J.T. 2004. Impact of a long asylum procedure on the prevalence of psychiatric disorders in Iraqi asylum seekers in the Netherlands. Journal of Nervous and Mental Disease 192,12: 843–852.

Laban C.J. Hurulean E. Attia A. 2014. Treatment of asylum seekers: resilience-oriented therapy and strategies (ROTS). Implication of study results into clinical practise. In: Golsabahi-Broclawski S. Özkan I. Broclawski A. (ed.) Transkulturelle Psychiatrie – Erfahrungen von Experten aus der EU. Berlin: LIT Verlag: 78–108.

Maier T. 2007. Sozialpsychiatrie und Sozialarbeit. In: Maier T. Schnyder U. (ed.)

Psychotherapie mit Folter- und Kriegsopfern. Ein praktisches Handbuch. Bern: Verlag Hans Huber: 117–129

Morgan C. Bhugra D. (ed.) 2010. Principles of Social Psychiatry. New-York: Willey-Blackwell.

Türkmen S. 2014. The Story in the Story of Gule. In: Golsabahi-Broclawski S. Özkan I. Broclawski A. (ed.) Transkulturelle Psychiatrie – Erfahrungen von Experten aus der EU. Berlin: LIT Verlag: 41–53.

Short CV

Malgorzata Symonowicz MA, studied Psychology and Migration Studies at Jagiellonian University in Krakow, Poland. She graduated her psychotherapeutic training at the Medical College of Jagiellonian University. She has professional experience as an anti-discrimination and diversity trainer. Since 2009, she is working with refugee women in the Berlin Center for Torture Victims. E-mail: m.symonowicz@bzfo.de

Mother-child multicultural group

Florence Faucherre, Julie Maillard

Introduction

The Unit Psy&Migrants of the psychiatry department of the University hospital of Lausanne is a specialized unit, created in 2010 to improve access to mental health care for all migrants. The unit is composed of a multidisciplinary team (psychiatrists, psychologists, social workers, researchers) and operate in several areas: formation and support to the professionals of the department, research, implementation of specific clinical settings. These settings are mainly dedicated to asylum seekers, as this population is especially vulnerable and faces multiple obstacles to psychiatric care services.

The mother-child multicultural group is one of the specific clinical settings that have been created by this unit.

Asylum context

Stressors potentially faced by asylum seekers are related to forced migration and resettlement. Many of them have suffered severe traumatic experiences in their homelands or during the flight (war, violence, poverty) and women are particularly vulnerable being often victims of sex and gender-based violence. Migration is also almost always correlated with a sudden and permanent separation of relatives and this loss may be difficult to deal with, inducing mental fragility.

Living conditions in the host country are an additional stress factor: precarious and uncertain residence status for a long time, deportation decisions, material and financial problems, unemployment and inactivity, living in collective centers, etc. Moreover, cultural and language barriers contribute to social isolation and adaptation stress. The cultural shift is significant for any migrant, but higher and more distressing for people coming from rural areas.

Mothering in the resettlement environment

For all women, pregnancy and motherhood are usually associated with mental fragility and often with anxiety and sadness and can lead to withdrawal and depression. Baby birth can also reactivate a trauma among some women, especially if they have been abused in the past.

Women seem to attach more importance to family knowledge and cultural rituals during pregnancy or at their first child's birth. The traditional practices should ideally match with those of the social environment to create a kind of holding function. However, in the migration context, those rituals or beliefs can't be shared with the host society. The local practices can as well sometimes seem strange or intrusive to the migrant mothers and the disciplinary practices may also be very different, in particular in regard to the use of physical discipline.

Furthermore, migrant women have often a limited social network and miss the proximity to relatives and the support they offered, and more generally the sense of shared responsibility that is part of child rearing in many cultures.

Finally, psychological vulnerability of the mothers (in case of depression or post traumatic stress disorder) can affect maternal care's capacity and the psychological development of their children: flashbacks, dissociation, sleep disturbance, irritability can disturb the mother-child link and not be compatible with the care requirements of a baby. Pacifying a child requires inner tranquillity that can be transmitted to the child but number of asylum seeker mothers doesn't have that tranquillity because of the tragic events they faced or because of the stress they're living in the host country.

Impact on mothers and children

This context of stress and multiple vulnerabilities can bring mental troubles among mothers and children. Among mothers, depression can be expressed as classic depressive symptomatology but also as somatic complaints, irritability with the baby, feelings of loneliness and isolation. The anxiety and post-traumatic stress disorders may often be expressed through worries about the baby and social demands. Studies have found that post-partum depressions are more frequent among migrant women.

Among children, behavioural disorders are often observed. The most common are hypertonic babies or hyperactive children (as if they attempt to wake up their mothers from depression). Developmental disorders can also appear across different domains: in emotional regulation, cognitive development, concentration problems, language delay and learning difficulties.

Limited access to mental health care system

Various factors limit access to health and social services for migrants and asylum seekers in general: discrimination, language and cultural barriers, lack of knowledge about the host country's resources and networks, unfamiliarity with medical practice. The lack of flexibility and cross-cultural skills in health institutions may also participate to limit this access.

In the field of mental health particularly, access to psychiatric and psychotherapeutic care is limited for asylum seekers and vulnerable migrants. Psychological difficulties are particularly insufficiently detected by migrant mothers and pregnant women and there is a lack of assessment, support and referral for psychiatric and psycho-social concerns. In this same context, the signs of developmental disorders in children are also poorly detected by paediatricians.

Migrant women are often reluctant to ask for help, either because they consider it stigmatizing, or because they minimize their children's developing psychological problems; uncertainty to seek care might also be due to mistrust or cultural inappropriateness of services. Finally, the potential gap between family/cultural knowledge and professional knowledge can also be a barrier to access to care.

Objectives

Part of the unfavourable health outcomes for the infants of ethnic minority women might be avoided by preventing inadequate infant care and psychological problems of the mothers. Different priorities and needs have been identified.

Prevention, assessment and support

First it is important to follow the women and children at risk and allow early appropriate intervention: support in parenting in a situation of isolation and insecurity, promoting the attachment process and screening mother-child bond's deficiency.

Transcultural and flexible approach

Transcultural and flexible approach is needed to improve access to care. It includes to overcome the language barriers and to acknowledge the expression of cultural representations of pregnancy, childbirth and mothering.

Multidisciplinary approach

Both psychological and social action are necessary to answer the multiple needs of these women.

Setting and results

Setting of the group

The group includes asylum seekers mothers, future mothers and children up to 5 years.

The group sessions take place every two weeks in a room within the center for asylum seekers. It is an open group and new women and their children can join the group anytime

Women are addressed by the primary care nurses or medical staff who have noted some psychological suffering and have suggested their patients to participate in the group.

There are three group leaders (a psychiatrist, a child psychologist and a social worker) and some translators (all participants speak their language and everything is translated)

Two rules are to be respected by all participants: confidentiality and a non judgemental attitude.

Participants and dynamic of the group

Women who have been participating until now are from sub-Saharan Africa, Eastern Europe, Middle East and Sri Lanka. Interpreters translate into Tigrigna, Tamil, Serbo-Croatian, Farsi, Albanian and Amharic. It is common that four of five languages are spoken simultaneously in the group. It should be noted that use of multiple interpreters complicates groupal interaction and slows down the exchanges.

Women are from mixed social backgrounds but many have a low level of education. They have mostly recently arrived in Switzerland and have a precarious legal status. Most participants face difficult living conditions, extreme isolation with low French proficiency and none is involved in any professional activity. The children are all less than 5 years old.

The geographical proximity of the group facilitates access to the treatment. The visibility of the group in the asylum seeker center has attracted other women who joined the group.

Patients' precarious immigration status causes frequent and unexpected departures from the center, related to transfers or deportation. These departures are also opportunities for talking about the women's anxiety due to the insecurity and instability of their living conditions.

During group session, women spontaneously intervene to express themselves, to speak to the animators or to respond to each other. Children are playing together and sometimes seeking contact with other mothers in the group. At the beginning of the session, the mothers are asked which concerns they have and what they want to speak about.

Other kind of exchanges take place during the sessions: sharing lullabies they sing to their babies, demonstration of massages or native techniques of care. Mothers also bring sometimes food and eat it together at the end of the session.

Benefits of group setting

Asylum seeker women are often suffering from social isolation and entering a therapeutic group gives them the possibility to develop relationships with other women and to reduce their loneliness. As this collective base creates a connection between family and social environment, it will help support maternal skills. Being part of a group gives also a feeling of belonging and the participation of pregnant women, babies and children in the group facilitates the integration of a new baby in the social group.

Secondly, the group provides participants with peer support, which is often more effective than one therapist's support. Sharing experiences and emotions is very rewarding. The collective recognition of having experienced violence and loss represents a key coping strategy. The participants also appreciate the warmth and the understanding of the other women and feel very comfortable in the group even when they are sad.

The group also facilitates the access to emotions, mental representations, narration and dreaming. When a woman is speaking in the group, she has to put words, chronology and sense on her thoughts in a narrative way and she has a public who is listening to her. Other participants often make comments, give advices and speak about their own experiences.

As in any group, many collective movements are observed which can be emphasized and commented. The most common movements that we can see are: identification, looking for similarities and linking, looking for differences and demarcation, splitting. We never saw movements of aggressiveness or exclusion. At most, we observed sometimes some rivalry and envy between the participants and these feelings could be spoken about. A group exclusively composed of women (and children) seems to offer a lot of freedom of speech, complicity and opportunities for identification.

Professional diversity

Multidisciplinary of the team answer the different objectives of the group at the interface of medical, psychological social and cultural fields.

Psychiatrist turns his attention to the expression of psychic suffering of women, the emergence of their difficulties and their elaboration. As main therapist, it is important for him to be trained in group therapy and to manage to support a participant in an individual way when necessary and, at the same time, keep in mind the whole group and its dynamics.

Child psychologist can identify signs of behaviour or developmental disorders, problems among babies and children, in the mother-babies link, and to give advices to mothers.

The presence of a social worker allows social concerns and daily stressors to be raised and processed in the group as the problems related to living conditions for the mothers and their children, accommodation, assistance, administrative status, take a lot of space in their expressed preoccupations.

Pesence of interpreters give mothers the opportunity to express themselves in their native language and ensures good communication and cultural metacommunication. Being familiar with both cultural contexts, they help promote trust and the link between host/origin cultures that can live in this group space.

Multidisciplinary and cross-cultural skills of the team help to establish the therapeutic alliance. Plurality of views reduces the risk of ethnocentrism linked to the Western practice and helps meeting the various concerns emerging in the group and identifying difficulties and resources on the different areas of our disciplines, (child psychology, psychiatry and social fields).

Moreover, multidisciplinary facilitate contacts with the networks of various disciplinary fields (child psychiatry, psychiatric, social) and allows to address some patients and / or their children to specialists for individual care.

Ethnic diversity

The group consists of women of very different ethnic groups. One of the aims of such a group is to give participants access to their cultural mental representations, to have the opportunity to talk about their traditional practices and to restore the meaning of these practices, valuing cultural resources.

The multiplicity of perspectives and opinions among the participants helps them to develop a cultural sensitivity, to decenter from their own beliefs, to broaden their outlook and to become more familiar with other customs. This also helps these women to build connections between many worlds that sometimes carry strong oppositions (health professions practise/family and cultural practise, for example) and to found mixed or new ways of parenting in this context of migration.

Main themes discussed

Child bearing/rearing: mothers speak a lot about their children, what they worry about and the difficulties to rear them being so distressed themselves. They also speak about their own practices, the way of carrying a baby, the way of feeding it, put it to sleep, the language they speak with, etc... Most of the women complain about the lack of an extended family and about the responsibility they have to take.

Living conditions: mothers living in a shelter frequently complain about the lack of comfort and hygiene for their babies, about noisy surroundings, bad smells. They also describe acts of racism against them or sometimes even relational difficulties with their compatriots. They are often speaking about their precarious residence status. Their low socio-economical status is also a common concern and the fact that they can't take a job, courses for qualifications or French lessons because they have no one to look after their children.

But they also discuss about the advantage to have a baby in Switzerland because of the sense of safety, the quality of health care and of the school system.

Troubles/ individual experiences: women of the group are very easily talking about feelings as sadness, dark thoughts, sleep disorders, nightmares, difficulty to focus, memory disorders. Regularly, pieces of individual stories are told within the discussions and this induces an atmosphere of shared confidence and privacy.

Cultural traditions: respective cultural traditions are expressed through sharing about rituals around pregnancy, childbirth, but also with witchcraft, beliefs about twins or infirmity. Differences and discordances can arise between the women.

Couple: discussion sometimes focuses on marriage, divorce, contraception, abortion, domestic violence, and also about the lack of a partner and being a single mother.

Conclusion

Proximity, flexibility and friendliness of the setting and close collaboration with the network give these women and their children the opportunity to access a therapeutic area and to receive care for their mental health troubles.

The setting helps creating links in a very large sense: social links and sharing between the mothers thanks to the group aspect; links between the professionals and the women and between the cultures of the host country and the country of origin thanks to the multicultural aspect; links with specialized mental health resources for mothers and children thanks to the multidisciplinary aspect which helps reducing reluctance and fears of consulting psychiatrists and psychologists.

Finally, the mix of various cultures of origin and various professional disciplines offers participants a kind of in-between space or a "transitional area" which is very useful for the process of decentering and facilitates the mental adaptation to a new diverse and complex cultural environment.

References

Mestre C. 2012. Face aux traumatismes maternels: soin et protection de la mère et de l'enfant. Manuel des psychotraumatismes :107–126.

Merry L.A. 2011. Refugee claimant women and barriers o health and social services post-birth. Revue canandienne de santé publique.

Fortin S. 2007. Néonatalité et constitution des savoirs en contexte migratoire: familles et services de santé. Enfances, familles, générations.

Levi M. 2014. Mothering in transition. Transcultural psychiatry51,4.

Moro M.R. 2011. Apaiser les enfants: une fonction parentale singulière et universelle. L'autre12,3.

Von Overbeck S. 2011. Tous parents, tous différents. L'autre12,3.

Goguikian B. 2011. Traumatisme chez des femmes en exil: dispositif de soin groupal. L'autre12,3.

Fenzing S. 1996. Alcoholism, a Contagious Disease. A Contribution towards an Anthropological Definition of Contagion. Culture, Medicine and Psychiatry20,4: 473–487.

Short CV

Unité Psy&Migrants, Département de psychiatrie, Centre Hospitalier Universitaire Vaud, Lausanne, Suisse

Unique experience of care on the Mental Health Day in the Siberian region of Russia

Gutkevich E.V., Lebedeva V.F., Bokhan N.A., Vladimirova S.V., Semke A.V.

Mental Health Research Institute, Tomsk, Russia

Life is *only* bearable when the *mind* and the *body* are in *harmony*,
and there is a natural *balance* between them,
and each has a natural respect for the other.
D. Lawrence

Abstract:

In the article relevant data on the World Mental Health Day, aims and tasks of actions carried out is provided. Data on the clinic of Federal State Budgetary Scientific Institution 'Mental Health Research Institute" (Tomsk, Russia) is presented where annually since 1993 Mental Health Days allow the population of the Siberian region accessing the psychiatric care. Results of carrying on the Mental Health Day for five years from two periods of development of the Russian society (2000–2003 and 2009, 2011), questioning of visitors of the clinic (2010–2011) are described in detail. Data on number of mental health care users, clinical characteristics of the revealed deviations in mental health, prevalence of mental disorders in the general population, attitude of patients and their relatives toward mental health problems was obtained which allows revealing main factors of mental disorders and developing preventive activities for improvement of quality of life of the population.

Keywords: Mental Health Day, mental health care users, screening-questionnaire, mental disorders, quality of life.

Introduction

In 1992, the World Federation for Mental Health has proposed to international community to carry on World Mental Health Day which provides unique possibilities: for the society – to make mental health a global priority and basic element of general health of the personality and its wellbeing; for business structures – to show social responsibility; for the general population – possibility of informing and training, involvement in this mass international movement, receiving the free professional specialised aid; for health care services – integration of process of treatment of mental disorders into activity of many institutions within health care reform.

In the Russian Federation on the basis of the clinic of Mental Health Research Institute the Mental Health Day has been carried on since 1993 [1, 2].The basic aims in medical work are as follows: approximation and accessibility of the specialised mental health care for the population; early detection, treatment and prevention of mental disorders using integration of extramural forms of psychiatric, psychotherapeutic and narcological service; introduction of novel methods of diagnostics and therapy, developed abroad and at leading Russian institutes, into practice; development of material resources and strengthening of personnel policy in the sphere of scientific research on maintenance and strengthening of mental health of the population in the regions of Siberia and Far East [3]. Activity of the clinic is completely conformable to the basic ideas and the purposes of activity of the World Federation for Mental Health therefore carrying on the Mental Health Day is a reasonable, logical and necessary action.

Objective

of this research was to analyse 20-year carrying on the Mental Health Day at Mental Health Research Institute, city of Tomsk, the Russian Federation, to assess relations between patients and doctors, to clarify viewpoints of doctors and patients regarding mental health problems, to find possibilities of collaboration of mental health professionals, mentally ill persons and their families in formation of anti-relapse behaviour in mental health service users.

Materials and methods – documentation on carrying on the Mental Health Day; data on number of visitors of the clinic of the Institute on Open Doors Days for 20 years from 1993 to 2012 (social-demographic, global-clinical and laboratory methods of examination). Data for 2000, 2002, and 2003 and for 2009, 2011 have been analysed. These periods were chosen, as reflecting the most general points during the periods of social and economic, political, organizational and legal development of the Russian society, the periods before economic crisis of 2008–2009 and after it. Express-questionnaire of persons, visiting the clinic of Mental Health Research Institute, Tomsk, Russia on World Mental Health Days 2010, 2011, 2012 was developed, distributed and analysed by user of mental health services, screening-questionnaire was carried out anonymously. Questions were answered by 14 persons of various ages, randomly selected by investigator. Respondents had to choose variants of answers for 4 questions:

1. What has encouraged you to come to clinic?
   a) Do you have your own mental health problems? b) Do you have relatives with mental health problems? c) Do you have friends with mental health problems? d) Just interesting.
2. Do you consider creation of site in the Internet for patients and their relatives as necessary?
3. Is there any need for organisation for patients and their relatives?
4. What assistance this organisation should render? a) Leisure activities b) Education of patients and their relatives c) Advocacy of rights of patients and relatives d) Provision with medications e) Other.

In 2011, 37 visitors answered the same questions. And that year sociodemographic data of respondents were collected: sex, age, education. In 2012, questions were answered by 51 persons of various ages, randomly selected by investigator. Respondents had to choose variants of answers for seven questions: 1. Your sex. 2. Your age. 3. Your education. 4. You place of living. 5. What mass media cover the topic of mental health best of all? 6. What do you think about people with mental health problems? 7. Are there persons with mental health problems among your relatives, friends or neighbours?

Results

Since 1993 annually in October, the Mental Health Research Institute carries on the Open Doors Day for population of the Tomsk Region, devoting this day a certain topic which is united by basic problems in the field of mental health. So quality, social-cultural, legal aspects of mental health were a priority in 1993–1995, 1998, 2007–2008; mental health of women – in 1996, of the unemployed persons – in 2000–2001, special attention was given to mental health of children and adolescents – 1997, 2002–2003 [4], of persons of elder age (1999) [5, 6], associations of mental and physical health, psychosomatic disorders determined 2004–2005, 2010 [7, 8]; 2006 and 2012 were devoted to risk of suicide and depressive mental disorders. Value of medical care, primary care, specialised and preventive services was covered in 2009, 2011 [9, 10].

At the initial stage of preparation, kit of documents is formed which includes announcements of the Mental Health Day for mass media; letters to sponsors and philanthropists. So, announcements of the Mental Health Day include information on time and venue of the Open Doors Day when doctors, researchers of the institute are ready to assist in diagnostics, treatment, psychotherapy, and psychocorrection, in the solution of personal, family, occupational problems which can cause low mood, onset of irritability, disturbances of sleep, heightened anxiety, depression, and headache. Information that "in the clinic, modern methods of research, such as encephalography, rheoencephalography, echoencephalography, ultrasonic diagnostics, computer brain mapping, medico-genetic consultation, immune status investigation, psychological consultation on family problems are provided" is obligatory mentioned. To sponsors and philanthropists, to social and responsible business structures the following information on the Mental Health Day is proposed. Along with written addresses, information on the Mental Health Day appears on TV and radio channels, newspapers, is placed in the Internet on the official site of the Institute.

In 2000, the Day was conducted on October 7 and has been devoted to mental health and labour, work. On this day, consultation was conducted by researchers and doctors with long-term experience; they rendered a free consultative and diagnostic help in issues of psychocorrection, psychotherapy, solution of occupational, personality, family and everyday problems. Medico-genetic consultation [11, 12], psychological testing, immune status investigation, encephalography, computer brain mapping, rheoencephalography, echoencephalography were carried out, if necessary. There were 135 visitors (105 women, 35 men). According to age patients were represented as follows: before 18 years – 5 persons, 19–25 years – 10 persons, 30–35 years – 60 persons, 50–60 years – 49 persons, more than 60 years – 11 persons. 19 % of visitors were elder persons, 4,1 % – disabled people, 12 % – schoolchildren, the group of the unemployed persons (about 22 %) was large. The consultative help has been rendered to 40 patients, 65 persons were referred for hospitalisation, 20 persons – for outpatient treatment. In the majority of patients (72 %) non-psychotic mental disorders were diagnosed, in 11,2 % – disorders caused by organic brain diseases, drug addiction – 4,6 %, alcoholism – 9,1 %, schizophrenia – 6,0 %. 4 patients received medico-genetic consultation, 2 – immunological investigation. The relevant causes of worsening the mental health were as follows: problems of social nature, financial difficulties, loneliness, lack of contacts with relatives, serious somatic-neurologic diseases, which severity is often conditioned by lack of possibility of adequate medication.

In 2002 (October 5), Day has been devoted to consequences of traumas and violence over children and adolescents. The relevance of the problem is conditioned by growth of mental disorders in persons of adolescent age in recent years which is influenced by social shocks of various nature and those arising in association with this adverse factor of the environment in family, at school, in society. On the Mental Health Day, 134 persons, including 2 families have visited the clinic. According to age, patients were distributed as follows: 15–18 years – 24 persons, 19–35 years – 42 persons, 35–45 years – 36 persons; 45–55 years – 12 persons; 55–65 years – 20 persons. 16 % of visitors were persons of elder age, 4,1 % – persons with mental disability, 24,7 % – unemployed persons, 18 % – schoolchildren. The consultative psychological-psychotherapeutic help was rendered to 38 patients (including 12 adolescents), 52 persons were referred for hospitalisation (including 10 adolescents), outpatient treatment was recommended to 30 persons (including 2 adolescents). Borderline mental disorders were diagnosed in most visitors of the clinic (76,25 %), drug addiction – 5,1 %, alcoholism – 8,0 %, schizophrenia – 4,1 %, personality disorders – 7,6 %. 2 patients received medico-genetic consultation, 5 – immunological investigation. Analysing worsening of mental health of adolescents, the following most relevant causes have been revealed: disturbances of interrelations in the family and with peers, emotional abuse and physical abuse of other persons, somatic and neurologic diseases.

The Mental Health Day on October 4, 2003 was also devoted to mental health of children and adolescents. On the Mental Health Day, 164 persons (including 21 families) have visited the clinic. According to age, patients were distributed as follows: 4–15 years – 44 persons, 15–18 years – 34 persons, 19–35 years – 19 persons, 35–60 years – 32 persons, also older than 60 years – 35 persons. The consultative-psychotherapeutic help was rendered to 30 patients (18 adolescents), 45 persons (21 adolescents) were referred for hospitalisation at the clinic, for outpatient treatment – 29 persons (2 adolescents).

In 2009, the World Mental Health Day has been devoted to the problem of mental health in system of primary care. Taking into account topic of the Mental Health Day and need for a complex clinical assessment of mental and physical status, in the clinic on the Open Doors Day consultations were conducted not only by psychiatrists, psychotherapists, addiction specialists, but also by doctors of other specialties – therapist, ophthalmologist, neurologist, immunologist, geneticist; the entire laboratory and diagnostic complex, services of functional and ultrasonic diagnostics functioned. There were 202 visitors (42 people more than in 2008), including 168 women, 34 men, 183 inhabitants of Tomsk, 19 persons from rural areas. In the analysis of age structure, it was revealed that unlike previous years when the age group "30–60 years" dominated, in 2009, 42 % of cases were persons aged more than 60 years. Accordingly, taking into account the social status pensioners, the unemployed persons due to age predominated, i.e. the persons seeking for medical help belonged mainly to most socially unprotected group. As analysis carried out showed, this contingent of visitors was in need for psychological-psychotherapeutic help to a lesser extent, and for consultative-therapeutic help of doctors of somatic profile to a major one. Of 202 persons, the consultative help was rendered to 123 persons, 42 persons were referred to psychiatric hospital, for outpatient treatment – 37 persons. In most patients (52 %) the condition was qualified as disorder of adaptive reactions conditioned by stressful events and life crises; in 12 % affective disorders were diagnosed, in 9,7 % – organic mental disorders, in 18 % – stress-related neurotic disorders, in 4 % – schizophrenia, 4,3 % – alcoholism. The main complaints presented by patients were dizziness – 31 %, sleeplessness – 30 %, headache – 15 %, low mood – 19 %, and somatised complaints without certain localisation – 30 %. Analysis of the causes of worsening of mental health, in particular, in persons of elder and old age revealed that problems of social nature, financial difficulties, loneliness, serious physical diseases which severity is conditioned in some cases by lack of possibility of appropriate medical care are the most relevant ones.

In 2010, the user of mental health services participated for the first time in conducting of Mental Health Day with questionnaire developed by her. 100 % of respondents of express-questionnaire have come to clinics for their mental health problems, among them 1 person (7 %) was a relative of person with mental health problems. 2 persons (14 %) had friends with mental health problems. One person said that it is just interesting for him. Patients and relatives need more information about mental health. They would like to know about available medication. Overwhelming number of respondents believed that establishment of site and organisation for mentally ill persons and relatives is necessary. Percent of negative answers was significantly lower and was explained by unwillingness to attract attention of other people. Organization of leisure-time would diversify life of patients and relatives. Of significance is advocacy of rights of patients and their relatives.

In 2011 (on October 8), the Mental Health Day has been devoted to the problem of funding of organisations of psychiatric help. The clinic was visited by 204 persons that were 15% more than in 2010, including 164 women, 40 men, 180 persons living in Tomsk and in rural areas – 24 persons. In the analysis of age structure it was established that in difference from previous years when the age group "30–55 years" dominated, in 2011

42 % were persons aged 30–60 years. Taking into account the social status, employees, persons, engaged in small business prevailed, more than 5 % were students, and 12 persons were adolescents. Of 204 persons the consultative help was rendered to 123 persons, 44 persons were referred to psychiatric hospital, 37 persons were referred for outpatient treatment. In most patients (52 %) their condition was qualified as disorder of adaptive reactions caused by stressful events and life crises; affective disorders were diagnosed in 12 %, organic mental disorders – in 9,7 %, in 18 % – neurotic stress-related disorders, in 4 % – schizophrenia, in 4,3 % – alcoholism. For verification of the diagnosis and assessment of leading symptom complex, physical-neurologic examination with investigation at room of functional and ultrasonic diagnostics was conducted for 25 patients, geneticist has examined 4 persons. In 2011, the user of mental health services took part in the Mental Health Day once again. She asked the same questions as in the year 2010 and collected sociodemographic data of respondents, which was as follows: Sex: women – 23 (62 %), men – 9 (24 %). 5 persons have not indicated their sex. Age: 36–74 years old. 5 persons have not indicated their age. Education: secondary school – 16 (43 %), high school – 14 (37 %), elementary school – 2 (5 %). Visitors participated in screening with caution.

In 2012, the author of above-mentioned questionnaire asked 7 questions and after thorough analysis of findings has concluded the following: regarding sex of participants it should be said that men were 0,1 % of the sample. The investigator has distinguished age characteristics of visitors. The first age group (22–48 years) and the third one (70–90 years) were somewhat little constituting 0,07 % and 0,05 %, respectively, second group (50–70 years) included 31,3 % of the sample. The rest respondents have not indicated their age. The third group has showed a new trend: interest of old people to their mental health and striving to have positive quality of life. Most visitors receive information about mental health problems from TV (58,9 %). Then news-papers, radio, books follow (51,1 %) and recently we may speak about increase of use of such mass medium as Internet (10 %). Use of Internet was typical for younger respondents. Answers to the sixth question have shown tolerance of respondents toward persons with mental health problems. Nobody said that such people should be kept at mental hospitals. 60,8 % of respondents have chosen the answer "mental illness is similar to every other illness (cardiovascular etc.)". 27,5 % of respondents consider mental patients with understanding. This shows changes in the society – decrease in stigmatization of mentally ill persons and decrease in self-stigmatization by these persons (majority has come because of their own problems). Such events are very important in life of the society. Analysis of screening-questionnaire has shown that social support is really needed by persons with mental health problems and it may be rendered by user-led organisations, need for which in Russia has not been still satisfied. Social support is important both for patients and their families because they are often isolated and hardly cope with challenge of poor mental health of ill family member.

Problems of social nature, loss of relatives, situations of family aspect, financial difficulties, loneliness, and chronic physical diseases were the most relevant causes worsening the mental health. Tables show detailed data (Tables 1, 2, 3, 4).

During comparison of two periods of observation it has been revealed that the number of visitors during the second period (after crisis of 2008) has increased 1,4-fold compared with number of the 2000th year. Number of visiting women has grown 1,1-fold. In both periods, persons of mature and elder age predominated. In three fourth of cases, non-psychotic mental disorders were diagnosed, among them – neurotic, affective, organic and personality disorders, drug addictions and alcoholism – in 15 % of cases, endogenous mental disorders – in 10 %. However, in the second period of observations, consultative, emergency assistance was rendered almost in two third of cases compared with the first period that may characterise severity of mental state of the visitors.

Discussion

Thus, need for carrying on the Mental Health Day is conditioned by the following: first, striving of psychiatrists to draw attention of the general public to issues of mental health and to cause interest in the problem discussed, formation of long-term activities for public mental health care, creation of the new attitude toward this problem, development of relevant interrelations between medical institutions and social departments; second, similar activities give the chance to all wishing persons, having problems in the state of mental health to receive a free, qualified help and, third, the analysis of the causes of conditionality of mental disorders, their nosological belonging allows carrying out rehabilitative activities more effectively, to develop preventive general medical programs focused on improvement of quality of life of the population. Speaking about prevention of mental health problems, attention should be paid also for secondary prevention, formation of anti-relapse behaviour, support of positive behavior and thought. The patients must have a need for absence of relapses. In order this need to appear, patients should be shown that they can feel well, think clearly if they receive appropriate psychopharmacological and psychotherapeutic treatment. They should be taught to trace their state, correctly assess it and understand what changes in their state may be caused by various interventions. Support of anti-relapse behaviour is an approach to removal of challenging behaviour and replacing it by prosocial skills.

Results of 20-year unique experience of carrying on the Mental Health Day in the Siberian region of Russia testify that services of mental health care and rendering of the specialised psychiatric help correspond to social and economic reforms occurring in Russia. Problems of identification of individual sensitivity to environmental factors, both internal, and external; international tolerance; latent narcotization and qualification of pre-illness forms of mental disorders in the population are thus solved. All this testifies to benefit of prospects of realisation of principles of predictive, preventive, translational medicine for strengthening the mental health of the population of the Siberian regions.

References

Lebedeva V.F., Yakutenok L.P. 2009. [About carrying on the Mental Health Day at Clinic of Mental Health Research Institute SB RAMSci]. Sibirskij vestnik psihiatrii i narkologii [Siberian Herald of Psychiatry and Addiction Psychiatry] 6: 117–118. (In Russ.).

Vladimirova S., Gutkevich E., Lebedeva V.F. 2010. Need for community-based services for mentally ill persons and their families. European Psychiatry 25, Suppl. 1: 729.

[The report on work of clinic of Federal State Budgetary Institution "Mental Health Research Institute" of Siberian Branch of the Russian Academy of Medical Sciences for 2013]. Edited by N. A. Bokhan. Tomsk, 2013; 36 p. (In Russ.).

Lebedeva V.F. 2012. Coping with psychosomatic problems of younger population in Siberia. 11th World Congress of World Association of Psychosocial Rehabilitation. Milan, Italy. 10–13 November 2012. Abstracts. P. 112.

Lebedeva V.F., Maltseva S.N. 2010. [Organization of psychiatric care for persons of gerontological age at outpatient stage]. Sibirskij vestnik psihiatrii i narkologii [Siberian Herald of Psychiatry and Addiction Psychiatry] 2: 43–45. (In Russ.)

Gutkevich E.V., Pavlova O.A., Lebedeva V.F. 2010. [Family of psychogeriatric patient (investigation of need for family-genetic prevention)]. [Ontogenetic aspects of mental health of the population: abstracts of scientific-practical conference (Omsk, April 19–20, 2010)]. Publishing House "Ivan Fedorov", Tomsk 52–54. (In Russ.).

Lebedeva V.F., Semke V.Ya., Yakutenok L.P. 2010. [Mental disorders in somatic diseases]. Publishing House "Ivan Fedorov", Tomsk 326 p. (In Russ.).

Lebedeva V.F., Belokrylova M.F., Garganeeva N.P., Semke V.Ya., Epanchintseva E.M., Redchits O.A., Kostin A.K., Lukiyanova E.V. 2011. [Peculiarities of medical rehabilitation of patients with non-psychotic mental disorders, associated with somatic diseases]. *Sibirskij vestnik psihiatrii i narkologii* [Siberian Herald of Psychiatry and Addiction Psychiatry] 4: 78–84. (In Russ.).

Gutkevich E.V. 2010. Mental health in families of Siberian region. Migration, next generations and the future of psychiatry. International Conference on Transcultural Psychiatry. Amsterdam, the Netherlands, 13–16 June 2010; 05.4.

Gutkevich E.V., Lebedeva V.F. 2013. [Organization of hierarchic system of genetic prevention of mental disorders in families as development of predictive-preventive and personalised medicine]. Sibirskij vestnik psihiatrii i narkologii of [Siberian Herald of Psychiatry and Addiction Psychiatry] 6: 33–40. (In Russ.).

Gutkevich E.V., Semke A.V., Semke V.Ya. 2011. [Family of mental patient in system of social co-ordinates (Russian research). Family-genetic crisis].Sibirskij vestnik psihiatrii i narkologii of [Siberian Herald of Psychiatry and Addiction Psychiatry] 1: 71–76. (In Russ.).

Vladimirova S., Gutkevich E., Lebedeva V. 2013. World Mental Health Day at community based services for mentally ill persons and their families. Romanian Journal of Psychiatry XV, Suppl. 1: 131.

Short CV

Elena V. Gutkevich – lead researcher of Endogenous Disorders Department of Federal State Budgetary Scientific Institution "Mental Health Research Institute", M.D., tel.: +7 382 2 723832, e-mail: gutkevich.elena@rambler.ru

Valentina F. Lebedeva – chief physician of the clinic of Federal State Budgetary Scientific Institution "Mental Health Research Institute", M.D., tel.: +7 382 2 724319, e-mail: redo@mail.tomsknet.ru

Nikolai A. Bokhan – director of Federal State Budgetary Scientific Institution "Mental Health Research Institute", M.D., Professor, tel.: +7 382 2 724015, e-mail: nikolay.bokhan.tomsk.russia@gmail.com

Svetlana V. Vladimirova – referent of director of Federal State Budgetary Scientific Institution "Mental Health Research Institute", tel.: +7 913 815 22 02, e-mail: niipzso@gmail.com

Arkady V. Semke – deputy director for research and clinical work of Federal State Budgetary Scientific Institution "Mental Health Research Institute", M.D., Professor, tel.: +7 382 2 724379, e-mail: asemke@mail.ru

List of tables

Table 1: Number of visitors of clinic on Mental Health Day

	2000	2002	2003	2009	2011
Number of visitors	135 persons (100 women and 35 men)	134 persons	164 persons	202 persons (168 women and 34 men)	204 persons (164 women and 40 men)

Table 2: Sociodemographic characteristics of visitors of clinic on Mental Health Day

	2000	2002	2003	2009	2011
Age group					
< 15 years			44 persons		
15–18 years			34 persons		
< 18 years	5 persons	24 persons			
19–25 years	10 persons				
19–35 years		42 persons	19 persons		
30–35 years	60 persons				
30–60 years					42%
35–45 years		36 persons			
35–60 years			32 persons		
45–55 years		12 persons			
50–60 years	49 persons				
55–65 years		20 persons			
> 60 years	11 persons		35 persons	42 %	
Social status					
Pensioners	19%	16%			
Persons with disability	4,1%	4,1%			
Students and schoolchildren	12%	18%			> 5%-students 12 schoolchildren
Unemployed persons	11%	24,7%			

Table 3: Outcome of encounter of visitor and specialist of clinic on Mental Health Day

	2000	2002	2003	2009	2011
Referral for inpatient treatment	65	52 (10 adolescents)	45 (21 adolescents)	42	44 adolescents
Consultation	40	38 (12 adolescents)	30 (18 adolescents)	123	123
Referral for outpatient treatment	20	30 (2 adolescents)	29 (2 adolescents)	37	37

Table 4: Nosological characteristics of visitors of clinic on Mental Health Day

	2000	2002	2009
Non-psychotic mental disorder	72 %	76,25%	52%
Organic mental disorder	11,2%		9,7%
Drug addiction	4,6%	5,1%	
Alcoholism	9,1%	8%	4,3%
Schizophrenia	6%	4,1%	4%
Disorder of mature personality		7,6%	
Affective disorders			12%
Neurotic disorders			18%

Polish people in Germany and the 'Matka Polka'

Dorothea von Kiedrowski

In Berlin lives a growing Polish community of circa 100,000 people. This fact brings new challenges also for psychotherapy, because – like my analysis of experiences of psychotherapists with a Polish migratory background will show – there are competitive myths, symbols and images of women and their lifestyles that can bring women into inner conflicts.

At the example of this group of psychotherapists, I directed my attention to the question whether therapists with a migratory background make the experience of foreignness in therapeutic settings with patients of the same cultural background. My master-thesis offered the frame for this analysis. For the analysis, I interviewed 5 of circa 14 registered psychotherapists with own practice in Berlin. Being mostly female the sample has been limited to women to keep it homogeneous.

The findings were analysed with Philipp Mayring's qualitative content-analysis and explained in the context of cultural imprint with the approaches of Cultural Studies. Mayring's qualitative content-analysis proved to be appropriate because of its open and descriptive approach. Both, the object of the research and the act of doing research – that the scientist is part of – are in an open process. The spoken is understood as a part of constructed social reality.

The five respondents were at the age of 46–56 years, work and live in Berlin and come from different psychological schools. They came as teenagers or young adults as late ethnic German repatriates (Spätaussiedler) from Poland to Germany. For the research, I randomised their names. Circa 10–90% of their patients have a Polish migratory background.

For the interviews, I chose the problem-centered interview that concentrates on the research problem and allows at the same time an open structure. The interviews have been held in German, because the psychotherapists as well as myself could express their thoughts more differentiated in German than in Polish.

How can the experience of foreignness be understood, especially when the actors seem to be familiar with the other's culture? The encyclopedia for Ethnopsychoanalysis begins its entry about cultural foreignness with a list of synonyms to characterise the foreign: "remote, distant, strange, different, unusual, unfamiliar, unknown, exotic"**1** Some antonyms on the other hand are "native, local, familiar, well-known". The foreign can release a discomfort, fear or fascination. As the psychotherapists can be understood as 'experts' of the Polish culture, it is something familiar that became foreign to them. With Freud it is about the familiar that is the Uncanny ("das Unheimliche")**2**

I came to the conclusion that the experience of foreignness originates in the first place from different ideas of values and norms – in this context, I examined especially different ideas of women's lifestyles. The image of women in Poland that the psychotherapists describe is diverse. They talk about working women and independent women but also about women being financially and emotionally dependent on their men or about women with difficulties to find their own way as foreigners in Germany. Besides, they use the notion 'Polish Mother' ('Matka Polka')**3** to describe a certain type of women:

"Here, I can say, it is distributed like, I don't know, 80 % very conformist women who live somehow this "Matka Polka" and a ..., recently I had one. It was very dramatic, as there was violence involved, and I told her clearly that she needs to take a stance, and this clear position of mine led to her not returning anymore." ("... da kann ich schon sagen, dass es so verteilt ist wie, ich weiß nicht, achtzig Prozent sehr angepasste Frauen, die dieses irgendwie "Matka Polka" leben und eine, neulich hatte ich eine, das war sehr dramatisch, weil eh es wirklich auch ehm Gewalt im Spiel war, und ich hab ihr ganz klar gesagt, eh dass sie sich positionieren muss, und diese klare Haltung von mir hat dazu geführt, dass sie nicht mehr gekommen ist, ne.") (A. Fischer)

Furthermore, the psychotherapists describe women with traits that can be seen as typical traits of a 'Polish Mother'. For example, those women would favour the welfare of the children and the family before their own needs and would make big sacrifices for their families. This trait although useful in some situations might also entail a low distinctive ability to perceive one's own emotions and needs. These women were mostly "conformist" ("angepasst") (A. Fischer) and had "not even a voice" ("nicht einmal eine Stimme") (B. Rosenberg). They would complain and would suffer from their own life situation, leaving their own needs behind: "Somehow struggling and fighting one's way through" ("irgendwie durchbeißen und durchschlagen") (A. Fischer). Another psychotherapist spoke about her sisters: "When I listen to my sisters, then one can say, in Poland it's just bad, yes, and this, I think, is too one-sided and this also annoys me" ("Wenn ich meine Schwestern höre, dann muss man sagen in Polen ist nur schlimm, ja, und das, denk ich mir, is zu einseitig und das stört mich auch, ne.") (D. Piotrowska)

It is conspicuous that the myth of the 'Polish Mother', or rather her traits, evoke emotions like anger, refusal and fear. Although the attributes of the 'Polish Mother', like caring, are interpreted as particularly positive, an uneasiness dominates the interviews while the mentioned qualities come up.

Thus, the questions seems to be relevant, why the symbol of the 'Polish Mother' and its traits evoke such emotions by emigrated women, even though they live in Germany since their youth or early adulthood. For that reason, I would like to cast a closer look at the question, who the 'Polish Mother' is, at her historico-cultural origins and the transitions of the myth, but also at current debates.

Origins in the 19th century

Thinking of the origin of the symbol of the 'Polish Mother', the poem of Adam Mickiewicz "To the Polish Mother" ("Do Matki Polki")**4** from 1830 is usually cited. How is the mother in this poem characterized? She is an unselfish woman who prepares her son for being a fighter and martyr for the sake of the Polish motherland. "Early tie up his hands with a chain,/ Tell him to harness to a wheelbarrow carriage,/ To not to go white in front of the katowski head/ And not burn seeing the rope" ("Wcześnie mu ręce okręcaj łancuchem,/ Do taczkowego każ zaprzęgać woza,/ By przed katowskim nie zbladnął obuchem/ Ani się spłonił na widok powroza")**5**

Women during the partition of Poland were expected to bear and raise the children in a patriotic manner, the teaching of the Polish language and culture as well as keeping the household, farming and doing business when the husbands went to fight. Women became all-round talents, something that often became overtaxing for them. The woman had to bear the different tasks and the emotional stress. Budrowska uses the term "the hero syndrom" ("syndrom bohaterski")**6** to describe a Polish mother who can carry every load. There is a strong connection between motherhood and the nation: Her devotion for the nation's well-being and her suffering have been idealised.

The role of a patriotic, unselfish and devoted woman is still alive in the collective memory of Polish people today. The function the myth had in the 20th century will be shown in the following.

The socialist era

The role model of a 'Polish Mother' appears in the Polish history especially in times of the loss of independence**7**; likewise, in the 20th century during the two World Wars but also during the socialism in the Polish People's Republic. The respondents, born and raised during that era, have been directly influenced by the role models of women at that time. The socialist elites used the symbol of the 'Polish Mother' for their purposes. The 'Polish socialist woman' should be as well mother as worker. Despite the professional equality with the men the women remained the main responsibles for the families and households. While the women's political influence remained low, they maintained their influence in the domestic sphere. Walczewska uses the term "the domestic matriarchy" ("matriarchat domowy) "**8** that defines a situation where a woman has the power over the family members. At those days, the women's task was quite laborious: to get the food in times of empty shops and long queues. Although this role of mothers has been full of self-denial, meant expenditure of time, a lot of work and exhaustion, women got recognition in this role. To maintain the apparent influence they did not let themselves help and preferred to infantilize the family members. Thus, a psychotherapist experienced her first time in Berlin as a student. "This has been this this role, that she has taken over and I really recognized, I came to Berlin and I didn't know, how to cook potatoes, yes." ("Ne, das war so diese, diese Rolle, die sie da übernommen hat und hab richtig gemerkt, ich kam nach Berlin und ich wusste nicht mal, wie man *Kartoffeln* kocht, ja.") (A. Fischer)

On the other hand, there have been the oppositional 'Polish Mothers' who put on the radio 'Free Europe' ('Wolna Europa') and printed and distributed leaflets. And again, these mothers lived in fear when their sons got arrested or injured in the protests against the socialist regime.

The post-socialist epoch, politics, the Church and the body

After the fall of the socialist regime, the first political regulation of the new 'Sejm' that has had a direct impact on women's freedom of decision-making has been the abortion law of 1993. Conservative parties like 'PIS' have taken up the myth of the 'Polish Mother' to construct a 'Polish' identity in a pluralistic Europe. Again, bearing a child is meant to be a duty towards the Polish nation. As Graff**9** claims, Poland's accession to the EU has revived certain fears to loose the national cohesion. Conservative circles therefore underline as specific 'Polish' features high moral standards, traditions and respect for the heterosexual family**10**. It has produced a public climate with huge protests against abortion and in-vitro-fertilisation as well as campaigns against contraception and homosexual partnerships. From the conservative point of view, the post-modern 'Polish Mother' should find her fulfilment in bearing and bringing up children. She also cares for other family members and manages the household, in which she feels indispensable. In a "manager of everyday life" ("menedżer życia codziennego")**11** one can see the parallel to the multiple traits and duties of women in the 19th century that have been already described.

There are parallels between the issues of conservative parties and the Catholic Church in Poland.

The myth of the 'Polish Mother' as a "post-romantic phantasm" ("postromantyczny fantazmat")**12** is often used in connection to Virgin Mary, who symbolizes maternity and devotion, purity and suffering for the sake of a higher cause. The Catholic Church picks up the symbol of the 'Polish Mother' to propagate a conservative family ideal. The original patriotic focus shifts to a woman's function as a mother. She gives birth and she saves the unborn live from the supporters of abortion. This Catholic-legal discourse is about a necessity to maintain a national tradition that is put in opposition to western role models. The respondents share a critical opinion about the Catholic Church in Poland. The Church is seen as "anti-women" ("frauenfeindlich") (A. Fischer) and would spread "mediocre" ("niveaulose") messages (D. Piotrowska), that many people would follow.

Poland's media challenge these days the traditional opinions of the Church and the conservative parties. In the broadcasting "The Polish Mother Feminist" ("Matka Polka Feministka") the radio station Trójka discusses questions as "Who rules today in Polish families? Is the father on paternity leave still a rarity? Is a marriage without children a family?" ("Kto dziś rządzi w polskiej rodzinie? Czy tato na wychowawczym to ciągle rzadkości? A małżeństwa, które nie mają dzieci, to też rodzina?")**13** Other subjects like "The new pill. Will Polish women get to like it?" (The "Nowa tabletka hormonalna. Czy Polki się przekonają? "are discussed in the morning-show "A question for breakfast" ("Pytanie na Śniadanie") on the TV channel WP tv**14** By doing so, the media promotes a reflection on partnership, sexuality and education. This represents a turning point in the history of the 'Polish Mother' as the ability to reflect her own needs and behaviours. As Kowalczyk claims in her analysis of Jałńska's artwork "SuperMother" ("Super Matka") that "Although the 'Super Mother' is not that far from the 'Polish Mother' – they differ in the degree of their consciousness of their location" ("chć Supermatka nie jest wcale tak bardzo odleła od Matki-Polki– rżni je przede wszystkim stopińświadomści własnegoulokowania.") **15** The 'new' mother or the "Super Mother "is able to look from a distance, is self-ironical and able to play with meanings.

The respondents recognized in their patients a rare consciousness of their living situations and a lacking ability of introspection. "Often, there is a demand for medicine or for advice, which means there is few consciousness what the work per se is about, to take one's life into your own hands and to try hard to work on it. ... So, there are high expectations to get something – be it by the State, by the family, by the church or by God." ("Es gibt auch häufig ein Verlangen nach Medikamenten oder nach Ratschlägen, also nach irgendetwas, was von außen eingegeben werden soll und dann soll es besser sein. Also, es gibt wenig Bewusstsein dafür, was die Arbeit an sich selbst bedeutet. ... Also, es gibt ne hohe Erwartung, etwas zu bekommen. Sei es eben vom Staat oder von der Familie oder von der Kirche oder von Gott.") (B. Rosenberg) The reaction of the psychotherapist to this phenomenon has been outraged and adversely. "Well, it is sometimes that difficult that I am already without hope. I could on the one hand fill my office with Polish patients alone, but on the other hand, it is very difficult to arrange the work with such patients." ("Also, das ist manchmal so schwierig, dass ich schon hoffnungslos bin. Ich könnte einerseits meine Praxis mit polnischen Patienten *alleine* füllen, andererseits aber eben ehm ist es ganz schwer diese Arbeit mit den Patienten zu installieren.") (B. Rosenberg)

Having a look at subjects that have not been mentioned by the respondents, one can note that the physicality, sexuality, the women's desire or female homosexual relationships have not been addressed. Interestingly, the myth of a 'Polish Mother' is an idea of a woman without a body**16** She denies herself and is not affected by "menstruation, giving birth under pain, [or] menopause" ("menstruacje, rodzenie w bólach, klimakterium")**17** Like the Virgin Mary she is expected to be beautiful, kind and pure ("Powinna być piękna, dobra i czysta")**18** The Immaculate Conception of Virgin Mary is also projected on the 'Polish Mother' – like Imbierowicz comments – nobody knows how the 'Polish Mother' came to her motherhood. Both moral examples suffer, but it is not a profane suffering. It just becomes visible for higher sacred causes. Mickiewicz writes in his poem that the 'Polish Mother' brings up her son to become a martyr – like Virgin Mary did

"The image of the Holy Family, well yes, well really, well before last century, as an image [has] to be destroyed." (Fischer, Z. 392–401) With the Virgin Mary is associated a 'holy' and intact image of the family. The impact of this role model can be seen in the importance of traditional family values in the Polish society. Boguszewski's results of a study about phenomena in marriage and family life shows: “Family values still take up the most important space, and the family bounds did not weaken relevantly for many years” (“Wartości rodzinne w deklaracjach Polaków zajmują wciąż najważniejsze miejsce, a więzi rodzinne w ich życiu od wielu lat nie ulegają istotnemu osłabieniu”).**19** Nevertheless the described changes and the competing images of women have apparent effects on family life. One can observe a shift from the traditional family to an economic community.**20**

Challenges in present days

The intention of this article has been to contribute an answer to the question, why the myth of the ‘Polish Mother’ evokes such emotions like uneasiness in psychotherapists with a Polish migratory background in Germany. For this purpose, I characterized the ‘Polish Mother’ and explained where the myth comes from regarding the historico-cultural origins and transitions of the myth and also the current debates. The historical retrospective has shown that the ‘Polish Mother’ is an ideal, whose traits like selflessness, devotion and purity are hardly attainable. Besides, it requires to suppress properties of the female body and its needs and limits. Furthermore, it became clear that female suffering fell silent for higher causes of the nation. The glorified but powerless women tended to exercise their power within their houses.

The myth of the ‘Polish Mother’ has its meaningful function, like Marcin Punpur claims. It integrates into a community, brings cohesion between the members through binding norms, values and behavioural patterns.**21** However in present days, the myth of the ‘Polish Mother’ is challenged by post-modern urges for individualism, secularism and consumption. Now individual needs are in the centre of attention. But this shift also leads to inner and family conflicts that are partly discussed in psychotherapeutic settings.

As it has been shown, the myth of the ‘Polish Mother’ is strongly anchored in the collective memory of Polish people. One reason for the strong emotions of the psychotherapists can be seen in the fact that they left their Polish ‘community’ and hence they do not participate any more in the Polish discourse about norms, values and behavioural patterns. Instead, they became members of a new 'community' with which they identify more. Their uneasiness can be understood as their conflicting memory of the myth of the 'Polish Mother' and its factual consequences for Polish women return as repressed impulses**22** This process is further stimulated by their migration. Hence, it remains a challenge for psychotherapists with a migratory background to remain non-judgemental. It could be helpful to take one's own cultural context into consideration and reflect one's own possibilities and limits leading through reflection to a "cultural adolescence" (kulturelle Adoleszenz")**23** This could be the way to stay cultural sensitive as psychotherapist**24**

Literature

1 H. Stubbe 2005. Lexikon der Ethnopsychologie und Transkulturellen Psychologie. Keyword "Transkulturelle Kinderpsychotherapie". Frankfurt am Main: 482–490.
2 S. Freud (1919) 1999. Das Unheimliche. In: Freud A. et. al. (ed.) Gesammelte Werke. Chronologisch geordnet. Vol. XII. Frankfurt am Main: 227–278.
3 In the following, I use the English term 'Polish Mother'.
4 All Polish and German citations are translated by myself.
5 A. Mickiewicz, Do Matki Polki. http://literat.ug.edu.pl/amwiersz/0055.htm, 21.08.2015.
6 B. Budrowska 2000. Macierzynstwo jako punkt zwrotny w zyciu kobiety. Wroclaw: 193.
7 Cf. A. Imbierowicz 2012. Matka Polka w defensywie? Przemiany mitu I jego wpłw na macierzynstwo polskich kobiet. Ogrody Nauk i Sztuk 2/2012: 431.
8 S. Walczewska 1999. Damy, rycerze i feministki. Kobiecy dyskurs emancypacyjny w Polsce. Kraków: 53.
9 A. Graff 2008. Rykoszetem. Rzecz o płci, seksualności i narodzie. Warszawa.
10 Ibid. 15–16.
11 A. Titkow, D. Duch-Krzystoszek, B. Budrowska 2004. Nieodplatna praca kobiet, mity, realia, perspektywy. Warszawa: 65.
12 M. Janion 1996. Kobiety i duchy innosci. Warszawa.
13 J. Mielewczyk, Matka Polka Feministka. https://www.polskieradio.pl/9/Audycja/8708, 12.08.2015.
14 B. Bieszczanian, Pytanie na Śniadanie. http://wp.tv/i,nowa-tabletka-hormonalna-czy-polki-sie-mid,1759146,cid,5050,klip.html?ticaid=61578aprzekonaja, 11.08.2015.

15 I. Kowalczyk 2003. Matka-Polka kontra supermatka? Ogrody Nauk i Sztuk 05/2003: 20.
16 Cf. Ibid.
17 Ibid. 17.
18 Ibid.
19 R. Boguszewski 2008. Kontrowersje wokol roznych zjawisk dotyczacych zycia malzenskiego I rodzinnego. Raport z badan CBOS. BS/54/2008. Warszawa: 20.
20 Cf. E. Illouz 2007. Gefühle in Zeiten des Kapitalismus. Frankfurt am Main.
21 Cf. M. Punpur, Logika Mitu. http://www.racjonalista.pl/kk.php/s,5337, 06.08.2015.
22 Cf. S. Freud (1919) 1999. Das Unheimliche. In: Freud A. et. al. (ed.) Gesammelte Werke. Chronologisch geordnet. Vol. XII. Frankfurt am Main: 227–278.
23 Cf. W. Machleidt 2013. Migration, Kultur und psychische Gesundheit. Dem Fremden begegnen. Stuttgart.
24 With thanks for a comment of a participant at the conference, who spotlighted the necessary differentiation between cultural competence and cultural sensitivity after my presentation.

Boguszewski R. 2008. Kontrowersje wokol roznych zjawisk dotyczacych zycia malzenskiego I rodzinnego. Raport z badan CBOS. BS/54/2008. Warszawa.
Budrowska B. 2000. Macierzyństwo jako punkt zwrotny w życiu kobiety. Wrocław: 193.
Choluj B. 2003. Die Situation der Frauen-NGO's in Polen an der Schwelle zum EU-Beitritt, in: Miethe I., Roth S. (eds.) Europas Töchter. Traditionen, Erwartungen und Strategien von Frauenbewegungen in Europa. Opladen: 203–224.
Freud S. (1919) 1999. Das Unheimliche. In: Freud A. et. al. (ed.) Gesammelte Werke. Chronologisch geordnet. Vol. XII. Frankfurt am Main: 227–278.
Graff A. 2008. Rykoszetem. Rzecz o płci, seksualności i narodzie. Warszawa.
Illouz E. 2007. Gefühle in Zeiten des Kapitalismus. Frankfurt am Main.
Imbierowicz A. 2012. Matka Polka w defensywie? Przemiany mitu I jego wpłw na macierzynstwo polskich kobiet. Ogrody Nauk i Sztuk 2/2012: 430–442, on www.ceeol.com.
Janion M. 1996. Kobiety i duchy innosci. Warszawa.
von Kiedrowski D. 2014. Konstruktionen des Fremden bei Psychotherapeutinnen in interkulturellen Psychotherapie-Settings in Bezug auf Geschlechterrollen. Masterarbeit am Lehrstuhl für Sprachgebrauch und Therapeutische Kommunikation im Fachbereich Interkulturelle Kommunikation, Europa-Universität Viadrina Frankfurt (Oder).

Kowalczyk I. 2003. Matka-Polka kontra supermatka? Ogrody Nauk i Sztuk 05/2003: 11–21, on www.ceeol.com

Machleidt W. 2013. Migration, Kultur und psychische Gesundheit. Dem Fremden begegnen. Stuttgart.

Punpur M. Logika Mitu. http://www.racjonalista.pl/kk.php/s,5337, access 06.08.2015.

Stubbe H. 2005. Lexikon der Ethnopsychologie und Transkulturellen Psychologie. Keyword "Transkulturelle Kinderpsychotherapie". Frankfurt am Main: 482–490.

Walczewska S. 1999. Damy, rycerze i feministki. Kobiecy dyskurs emancypacyjny w Polsce. Kraków.

Websites

Mielewczyk J. Matka Polka Feministka. https://www.polskieradio.pl/9/Audycja/8708, access 12.08.2015.

Bieszczanian B. Pytanie na Sniadanie http://wp.tv/i,nowa-tabletka-hormonalna-czy-polki-siemid,1759146,cid,5050,klip.html?ticaid=61578aprzekonaja, access 11.08.2015.

Short CV

Dorothea von Kiedrowski, born 1982 in Toruń (Poland) has emigrated to Germany at the age of seven. After a Diploma in Fine Arts she obtained a M.A. in Intercultural Communication Studies from European University Viadrina in Frankfurt (Oder). Her main interests are phenomena of the perception of others in the Polish and German culture.

Attempted self – "pervasive refusal syndrome"

M. Río Benito and M.-C. Dubois

We would like to share with you one of the complex clinical situation we have received in our consultation and to discuss about the philosophy of our therapeutic approach. We could name it as:

A father prisoner of his shame, a child prisoner inside his body, a mother prisoner of her husband and son's illnesses, the therapists prisoners of their powerlessness?

Appartenances was born in 1993, in response to the wave of immigrants and asylum seekers from the Balkans. It has different departments:

- The Psychotherapeutic Service for Migrants
- Community Interpreters Department
- Community Services: Women's Centre and Mozaïk Psycho Social Centre
- Training Department

Appartenances's mission is:

- To promote the wellbeing and the independence of migrant people
- To facilitate integration in the host society
- To answer to the different psychological and social needs of migrant people with a holistic psychosocial, multidisciplinary, culturally sensitive approach, working with people's coping strategies and resources.

Clinical situation

It is a family clinical case. They come from Armenia: the father is 38 years old, the mother, 43 and their only child is 15.

The parents (both Christian) get married against her parents' will (madam's family did not agree because their daughter was older than her groom). Madam had several miscarriages before and after their son's birth.

The father was in the army to fight the Azeri's, but was injured very soon. As he could not fight, he felt powerless and ashamed.

He was working as a hawker in the market when a man insulted his wife and, as a reaction, our patient responded very aggressively. He was imprisoned for a year. During this period he was raped by 3 persons. This rape was recorded with a telephone. Our patient thinks that this rape was related to the aggression in the market and that was organised by the victim's family. He was also victim of a financial blackmail. He drank a lot of alcohol and tried to commit suicide with an overdose of medicaments in prison and once he was outside the prison, by hanging himself. During his time in prison, his son did not know why he could not see his father.

In order to escape further violence and retaliation, the family came to Switzerland in February 2012 and claimed asylum. At the beginning, the father, who developed psychotic traumatic symptoms, was treated at the Psychiatry Department and his mental health improved. The son was well integrated with good results at school.

Unfortunately, their asylum claim was rejected and when the father received the news, in March 2013, he poured alcohol over himself in front of his wife and their son with the intention to immolate himself. Fortunately, he could not do it thanks to police help. He was hospitalised for several weeks in a non – voluntary admission.

After this extremely traumatic episode, the son started developing psychiatric symptoms: sadness, enuresis, anorexia.

In order to find safety and security they left Switzerland for Sweden in August 2013. The son was soon hospitalised because he developed a pervasive refusal syndrome: he stopped eating, moving, speaking. Despite that, the family was sent back to Switzerland in October 2013. This time, they were only allocated a room in a centre for asylum seekers, whereas before they had a flat. The child was hospitalised in Lausanne.

I started the therapy with the father in December 2013, and my colleague Marie Claire Dubois treated the mother later for a short time. This woman was highly distressed by her son's illness (she spent all the time in the hospital near her son) and the situation of her husband.

All the therapeutic sessions with the father and the mother were with an Armenian interpreter. At my first session with the father, he clearly stated that he didn't want to speak about his traumatic past, but he agreed that all the clinical information be sent to us by his former psychiatrist. I focused the intervention in the present, in the here and now:

- His son suffering, hospitalised for months
- His difficulty to find his role in the family
- His tendency to drink a lot again
- His anger against the Swiss authorities who would not give them a flat where their son could come the week ends when he was able to be in a wheel chair)

My aim in the sessions was to diminish the risk of suicide, to support my patient in his parenting role, to listen to his social needs and to try to enhance his feelings of security. At the same time I was in contact with his son's psychiatric network and I could participate in meetings with both parents. I consider these two meetings as two important moments for the clinical evolution of the family:

1. The first meeting, in January 2014, was in the general hospital where the son was hospitalised since the family returned to Switzerland from Sweden. After this meeting the family's social assistant in the hospital coordinated all their social requests. Communication between the father and the network improved when the hospital changed the interpreter. The first interpreter translated from French into Russian (a language that only the mother understands and speaks fluently, but not the father). After this meeting, with the new interpreter, the father found better his place caring about his son.
2. The second meeting, in June 2014, was in the psychiatric ward for adolescents where the son was moved a few months later. I prepared this meeting with my patient with the objective to inform the son's therapists about the traumatic events that this family had lived. My patient asked me to be his voice in front of them, explaining the relationship between his son's state and his state. At the end of the meeting the son came in his wheel chair. I introduced myself to him as the psychiatrist who took care of his father, encouraging him to care about himself. The son's therapists informed all the family about an early discharge from the hospital.

The father participates to ergo therapy sessions at Embellimur, an Association of social ergo therapy that looks for enhancing the capacities of participants.

In March 2015 I had my last interview with my patient in Appartenances. He came to tell me that the Swiss authorities had given them a flat in Lausanne and that his son had started to walk a few days after his return to school. He offered to me a last gift in this last day: He thanked me for my help during this time and told me that he was ready to work on his traumatic past with an Armenian psychiatrist (former colleague of our association).

By this follow up in our psychotherapeutic service for migrants we would like to show some of the principles of our philosophy when treating asylum seekers

1. Social conditions, in rich countries as well, are related to the health status of persons. Asylum seekers suffer relative poverty.
2. Asylum seekers ask the therapists practical help for improving their lives and the lives of their families. Writing medical reports is one of our activities that tries to help them. Communicate with the network on behalf of them is another one. Referring them to psycho social settings is another way to help them (inside our association or outside).
3. Asylum seekers expect us to witness their suffering. The medical report has in part this function.
4. Asylum seekers also expect us to alleviate their symptoms. Solution Focused Psycho traumatology gives to us useful clues to treat symptoms. Each therapist feels free to use the approach which is more familiar with.
5. We usually are three in the consultation: the patient, the interpreter (co therapist), and the therapist. The expert of patients' life and of patient's needs is the patient. The interpreter and the therapist offer their general knowledge and experience to help this particular patient by creating a relationship (respect and recognition are the bases of this therapeutic relationship).

References

Some of the authors who help me

1. Nunn, Lask, Owen. Pervasive Refusal Syndrome (PRS) 21 years on: a re-conceptualisation and a renaming. Eur Child Adolesc Psychiatry (2014) 23:163–172
2. Dellucci Hélène. Psycho traumatologie centrée compétences. Thérapie Familiale 2014 / 2 (vol 35)
3. Social Determinants of Health. The Solid Facts. Marmot & Wilkinson. Second Edition. WHO 2003
4. La migration comme méthaphore. Jean-Claude Métraux. Ed. La Dispute. 2011
5. http://embellimur.org

Short CV

M. Río Benito (psychiatrist and psychotherapist) and M.-C. Dubois (psychologist). Psychotherapeutic Service for Migrants, Appartenances Association. Lausanne, Switzerland

Opowieści transkulturowe jako narzędzie pracy psychiatry w codziennej praktyce klinicznej. Transcultural Stories as Techniques of Psychotherapy in Everyday Practice

Ewa Dobiala, MD (Poland)

Polskie Stowarzyszenie Rozwoju Psychoterapii
Wrocławskie Centrum Psychoterapii Pozytywnej

Współczesny świat doświadcza migracji międzynarodowych na skalę dotychczas niespotykaną. Na naszych oczach rośnie potrzeba jednostki zarówno do wewnętrznej integracji myśli i uczuć jak i do rozpoznania własnych wartości, kultury rodziny pochodzenia, zinternalizowanych modelów wymiarowania (pojęcie z PPT). Konsekwencją tych przemian może stać się zarówno rozwój człowieka jak i doświadczanie różnych zespołów objawowych. Zmiany kulturowe, które zachodzą w funkcjonowaniu społeczeństw znajdują swoje odzwierciedlenie w treściach wnoszonych do gabinetów lekarskich. Staje się to jedną z przyczyn obserwowanego w ostatnim czasie wzrostu zgłoszeń zarówno do gabinetów lekarzy rodzinnych jak i do psychiatrów i psychoterapeutów osób z doświadczeniem migracji międzynarodowej z różnorodnymi objawami psychosomatycznymi, lękowymi, afektywnymi i in.

Rola języka w psychiatrii transkulturowej. The role of language in transcultural psychiatry.

Jednym z podstawowych wyzwań przed którym stajemy w roli "pomagaczy" jest język. Paradoksalnie trudność ta pojawia się nie tylko w odniesieniu do pacjentów, dla których język ojczysty jest obcy terapeucie. Pojęcia medyczne, psychiatryczne potrafią być równie hermetyczne i lękotwórcze jak brzmienie zupełnie nieznanego dialektu.

"Pewien król zwołał dwór, by poddać jego członków próbie. Wokół tronu zebrali się najmądrzejsi i najbardziej znaczący obywatele w królestwie.

– Słuchajcie dostojnicy i uczeni- powiedział- zebrałem was tutaj, ponieważ potrzebna mi jest wasza pomoc"

Następnie zaprowadził ich do olbrzymich drzwi, większych niż kiedykolwiek widziano

– Oto widzicie największe i najcięższe drzwi w królestwie. Kto z was je otworzy? – zapytał król.

Niektórzy z obecnych przecząco pokręcili głowami. Inni, uważni za uczonych przyjrzeli się drzwiom nieco dokładniej, lecz przyznali w końcu, że nie zdołają ich poruszyć. Usłyszawszy opinię uczonych, także pozostali zgodzili się, iż zadanie jest niewykonalne.

Tylko wezyr, jedyny spośród obecnych, podszedł bliżej drzwi, obejrzał je dokładnie, a także dotykał w różnych miejscach, aż wreszcie pociągnął je mocno i zdecydowanie. I podwoje się otwarły. Okazało się bowiem, że nie tyko nie były zamknięte, ale cały czas pozostawały lekko uchylone i że trzeba było jedynie chęci, śmiałości i zdecydowanego działania, aby wypełnić zadanie…"

Metafora jako odwieczny sposób komunikacji. Metaphor as one of the oldest way of communication.

Ludzkość wykształciła setki różnych języków i tysiące ich odmian. Każdy z nich wymaga znajomości leksykalnej, zasad gramatycznych itd. Jednakże na przestrzeni wieków wykształcił się jeszcze jeden model przekazywania informacji- metafora. Obecna jest ona we wszystkich kulturach będąc uniwersalnym sposobem komunikacji. Odnajdujemy ją w bajkach, opowieściach, anegdotach, mitach, przysłowiach i przypowieściach biblijnych.

Rola bajek i opowieści w naszej kulturze. The role of fairly tales and stories in our culture.

O roli bajek i opowieści w kulturze człowieka powiedziano i napisano już bardzo wiele. Nie ulega wątpliwości, że jest to bardzo skuteczna forma porozumiewania się. Jest użyteczna w argumentowaniu, sugerowaniu znaczeń czy prowokowaniu refleksji. Może stać się bezpiecznym obszarem dla przekazu istotnych informacji jednocześnie bawiąc i przytrzymując uwagę.

Użyteczność metafory w procesie terapeutycznym. The usefulness of metaphors in the therapeutic process.

Język wyjaśnień, profesjonalizmów często prowadzi do izolacji i fragmentacji, język metaforyczny ma moc syntetyzowania i łączenia.

Znaczenie metafory jest odbierane na dwóch poziomach. Niesie ze sobą znaczenie dosłowne, które jest w prosty sposób wyłapywane na poziomie świadomym oraz warstwę symboliczną, odbieraną na poziomie zarówno świadomym jak i nieświadomym.

Ta właściwość metafory czyni ją niezwykle użytecznym narzędziem w procesie terapeutycznym.

Świadome używanie tego narzędzia w pracy z pacjentem pozwala na uaktywnianie doświadczeń, uczuć, wyobrażeń w adekwatnym momencie terapii. Bajki, opowieści są naszym dziedzictwem kulturowym. Ich różnorodność stanowi o naszym bogactwie. W ich symbolicznej treści pacjent może odnaleźć odzwierciedlenie własnej sytuacji i przeżyć. Rozumiane i odbierane bardzo indywidualnie znaczenie potrafi otwierać nowe możliwości, przeformułowywać, a także modelować nowe zachowania. Metafora może odgrywać też – niezwykle istotną w psychiatrii transkulturowej- rolę mediacyjną. Dosłowne rozumienie warstwy znaczeniowej zazwyczaj ma drugorzędną rolę względem uruchamianego wewnętrznie procesu wyobrażeniowego, emocji, poruszenia.

Metaforyczny przekaz poruszając wyobraźnię pacjenta może obudzić nagłe zrozumienie lub zapoczątkować stopniowy proces uczenia. Jest zwykle bardziej zajmujący niż bezpośrednie wyrażanie jakiejś myśli. Staje się bardzo skutecznym i bezpiecznym narzędziem w budowaniu relacji. Znaczenia, komunikaty wyrażane pośrednio odbierane są jako zdecydowanie mniej zagrażające i otwierają przestrzeń do bardzo indywidualnego odbioru i odnalezienia własnego znaczenia. Elastyczność i wielopoziomowość znaczeniowa opowieści pozwala przekazywać różne komunikaty jednocześnie: rozwiązania, opinie, informacje, możliwości, nowe punkty widzenia.

Kliniczne zastosowanie metafory. The clinical use of metaphor.

Znaczna użyteczność metafory w procesie terapeutycznym pozwala zrozumieć jej szerokie kliniczne zastosowanie.

Jest to narzędzie, które w zależności od etapu terapii, może być wykorzystywane zarówno do pracy nad motywacją, budowaniem "ego" czy do kontrolowania relacji terapeutycznej. Jest niezwykle skuteczne w kontaktowaniu i asocjacji pacjenta z jego zasobami, wartościami, czy zinternalizowanymi modelami wymiarowania. Znajduje swoje wykorzystanie w pracy nad desensytyzacją czy integracją stanów "ego".

Kryteria sensowności użycia metafory w psychoterapii. Criteria for the use of metaphors in psychotherapy.

Rozważając użycie bajek, przypowieści, anegdot w terapii dobrze uwzględnić kilka aspektów przynależnych zarówno dla pacjenta jak i terapeuty. Warto reflektować sytuacje kliniczną oraz treści, które terapeuta chciałby na tym etapie terapii przekazać. Pomocne bywa rozpoznanie sposobu odpowiedzi pacjenta na bezpośrednią i metaforyczną formę komunikacji. Po stronie terapeuty kryteriami sensowności jest zarówno szkoła psychoterapeutyczna, w koncepcji której pracuje jak i jego indywidualne doświadczenie i preferencje. Komunikacja metaforyczna jest jednym z podstawowych narzędzi Psychoterapii Pozytywnej Peseschkiana i Hipnoterapii

Ericksonowskiej. Znajduje też swoje miejsce w terapiach systemowych, strategicznych i in.. Poczucie pewności terapeuty i pewna swoboda w tym języku komunikacji warunkują skuteczność posługiwania się tą techniką w pracy z pacjentem. Dorastamy w kulturze, gdzie opowieści zwyczajowo używa się do sugerowania znaczeń, przedstawiania argumentów, przekazywania informacji, perswadowania, prowokowania refleksji, rozśmieszania i zabawiania. Jest to dziedzictwo, które wyposaża nas w model tej bardzo skutecznej metody porozumiewania się.Te drzwi do przestrzeni, w której możemy się spotkać bez względu na język, narodowość, wykształcenie, historię czy religię być może od wieków pozostają więc otwarte.

Transkulturowa Psychoterapia Pozytywna (prof. Peseschkian). Tancultural Positive Psychotherapy (prof. Peseschkian).

Jedną ze szkół psychoterapeutycznych traktujących metaforę jako podstawowe narzędzie i znajdującą swoje zastosowanie w codziennej pracy w psychiatrii transkulturowej jest Psychoterapia Pozytywna. Twórcą i popularyzatorem podejścia był prof. Peseschkian, klinicysta, psychiatra, neurolog pochodzenia irańskiego, pracujący i żyjący w Niemczech. Opracowana przez niego metoda (1968 r.) jest terapią krótkoterminową integrującą myślenie psychodynamiczne i poznawczo-behawioralne z jednoczesnym odwołaniem się do humanistycznej wizji człowieka, koncepcji salutogenezy oraz doświadczeń transkulturowych. Narodowe Instytuty Psychoterapii Pozytywnej są aktualnie obecne w 26 krajach. Szkolenia w tej modalności zakończyło dziesiątki tysięcy specjalistów: lekarzy, psychiatrów, psychologów, pedagogów z różnych zakątków świata. Ich wspólna praca i reflektowanie dynamiki intra- i interpsychicznej odpowiedzi człowieka na jego losowe sytuacje w dobie tak nasilonej migracji stanowi kolejne kroki ku humanizacji spojrzenia na wyzwania psychiatrii transkulturowej z jednoczesnym poszanowaniem empirycznego dorobku zarówno medycyny, psychiatrii jak i psychologii. W Polsce szkolenia z Psychoterapii Pozytywnej odbywają się od 2011 roku. Centrum Psychoterapii Pozytywnej mieści się we Wrocławiu.

Piśmiennictwo
References

Opowieści orientalne w psychoterapii pozytywnej. Kupiec i papuga. N Peseschkian, Warszawa, 2014

Positive Psychotherapy- Theory and Practice of new Method, N. Peseschkian, Fischer TB, Frankfurt

Metafory w psychoterapii. P. Barker, Gdańsk 2000

Short CV

Ewa Dobiala, MD (Poland)
Polskie Stowarzyszenie ozwoju Psychoterapii
Wrocławskie Centrum Psychoterapii Pozytywnej